ETHICAL
PRACTICE
IN EVERYDAY
HEALTH CARE

ETHICAL PRACTICE
IN EVERYDAY HEALTH CARE

E.R. WALROND

University of the West Indies Press
Jamaica ● Barbados ● Trinidad and Tobago

University of the West Indies Press
1A Aqueduct Flats   Mona
Kingston 7   Jamaica
www.uwipress.com

09 08 07 06 05   5 4 3 2 1

CATALOGUING IN PUBLICATION DATA

Walrond, E.R.
Ethical practice in everyday health care / E.R. Walrond

p. cm.

Includes bibliographical references.

ISBN: 976-640-164-0

1. Medical ethics – Study and teaching. 2. Medical care – Law and
legislation. 3. Confidential communication – Physicians.
4. Medical ethics – Case studies. I. Title.

R724.W35 2005   174.2

Book and cover design by Robert Harris.
E-mail: roberth@cwjamaica.com

Set in Veracity 10/14.5 x 32

Printed in the United States of America.

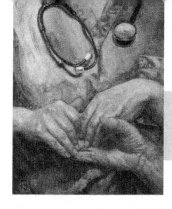

Contents

Preface

The public expects members of the medical profession to conduct themselves according to the terms of the Hippocratic oath, yet few physicians and virtually no laypersons know what is in that oath. For the oath to reach beyond its symbolic importance, ethical conduct must be learned and practised. There are many texts on the practice of medicine, surgery and all of the related disciplines, yet one is hard pressed to find anything on ethical practice in any of them.

Scholarly texts on ethics tend to deal with the landmark issues and dilemmas that have occurred within particular jurisdictions or religions. This book is intended as a student-friendly text that seeks not to turn students into ethics scholars but to provide them with a practical guide to ethical conduct in everyday medical practice. Ethics is taught in various ways; in this book exercises and discussion are provided for each area addressed. The exercises are a tool to stimulate thought about ethical conduct, which I believe is more valuable than simply memorizing appropriate responses to given situations.

Two case studies demonstrate that apparently simple ethical issues can be multifaceted and may require the consideration of a number of angles. They also illustrate that dealing with problems that arise in practice is a process rather than an event.

The book demonstrates that ethical conduct is not always a matter of black and white or right and wrong. Rather than attempting to prescribe for every situation, I suggest principles that can be used to solve problems and to conduct oneself ethically as a medical professional.

Acknowledgements

I acknowledge with thanks all of those colleagues who have read the manuscript and encouraged me to get it published. In particular, I would like to thank the colleague who suggested that some student exercises should be added, and one of my patients, who took an interest in what I was writing and offered literary comments on the text.

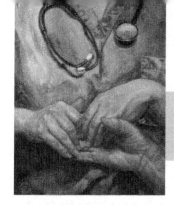

CHAPTER 1

Ethical Practices in Health Care

The *Shorter Oxford English Dictionary* defines ethics as *moral philosophy or principles*. More expansive definitions usually raise further questions: What or whose morals? Which or whose philosophy? and Where are the principles to be found? A search for the definition of morals can seldom be divorced from reference to religion. However, religions vary on what is right or wrong, and religious differences can extend into the branches of one religion and may even depend on the context within a particular religion. To cite a familiar example, the use of contraceptives is considered morally wrong in the Roman Catholic Church but not in many other Christian denominations [see Exercise 1].

Ethics can therefore be difficult to define precisely and should be looked at as a code of conduct that will change from time to time as society and the professions reach a consensus on what actions are right and wrong. It is generally agreed among writers on medical ethics that ethical conduct in health-care practice is based on the principles of *beneficence, non-maleficence, autonomy* and *justice* (Gracia 1990; Sass 1990).

Beneficence – to do good

The anticipated good of any therapy must be defined. The four goals of good health care are to relieve symptoms, cure disease, prolong life and improve the quality of life. One hopes that these four goals will coalesce, but they do not necessarily do so. When they do not, one or another factor may carry more weight in the thinking of both the health-care professional in offering advice and the patient or relative in giving consent to therapy.

Non-maleficence – to do no harm

The perception of potential harm that can be done will depend on whether you are the doctor, the patient, the relatives or even the society. For example, a surgeon may have the attitude that if a patient is likely to die, trying a risky procedure with a small possibility of success will do no harm. This conjures up the saying "The operation was successful but the patient died." Some patients or relatives may share the view that a chance at life is worth the risk, but many do not, for if the procedure fails, they consider that harm was done by the therapist or the therapy.

Autonomy – the patient's right to decide

Patients have the right to consent to anything that is done to them, including examination, investigation and therapy. Autonomy implies a broad concept of consent that requires that patients be given all available information. Although patients may trust their practitioner and say "You know best", this should not be construed as giving the practitioner the right to make decisions for the patient.

Justice

The concept of justice in health care is relevant not only to a patient's access to the courts should something go amiss but also to the broader concept of patients' rights. Patients have a right to access to care and a right to have their religious and cultural values respected. Justice is also about equity, where access to care is not determined solely by the ability to pay, social status or even race.

Ethical issues in health-care practice are currently being raised with a frequency that demands that closer attention should be paid to this matter. It is sometimes difficult, however, to find ethical issues clearly articulated in everyday practice, for those who raise them and those who respond may start from different understandings of what is ethical. Decisions about doing what is right or good as opposed to doing wrong or harm are often based on firmly held individual and societal beliefs grounded in different religious traditions. What is perceived to be correct action not only varies from person to person but can vary between disciplines and professions and in societies, so that there are often no clear-cut answers to certain questions. It is therefore important to look at ethical questions from a multidisciplinary point of view and, through discussion and consensus, provide guidance in those areas that are not clear. By the same token, it is vital that health-care providers and the society at large know what ethical conduct is agreed upon so that conflicts in health-care practice may be recognized, scrutinized and, where possible, resolved. Health practitioners should familiarize themselves with whatever code of ethics governs their profession in their jurisdiction.

Ethics and religion

The most sensitive areas of possible ethical conflict in health care are related to religious beliefs, in particular beliefs about life and its preservation, the interpretation of religious texts as they relate to medical treatments, and, in some instances, religious rituals that have medical implications. Abortion remains an area of unresolved conflict, but in most jurisdictions its practice is guided by specific legislation. When religious beliefs conflict with *standard* medical practice, the patient's religion should be respected – unless those beliefs conflict with the law. For example, the right of a Jehovah's Witness to refuse blood transfusion should be respected, whereas a Rastafarian's claim of the right to use marijuana cannot be entertained in jurisdictions where its use remains illegal. A Muslim may have to forgo a religious objection to post-mortems to satisfy the law in the case of accidental or sudden unexplained death.

As regards religious rituals with medical implications, circumcision of Jewish and Muslim male infants is a recognized and accepted practice, whereas female circumcision, practised in some African cultures, is frowned upon and considered harmful outside of those cultures. Many cultural practices are intertwined with religion; when they are encountered during the course of health care, they should be respected wherever possible. A Muslim may hold strong views about the physical examination of one gender by the other. Hindus have strong religious objections to eating beef, whereas various religions prohibit the eating of pork. These practices have implications for catering to the needs of hospitalized patients. Modes of dress or grooming may have a religious basis, such as the Muslim chador and the Rastafarian's dreadlocks (the latter may appear to some health-care workers to be unhygienic).

Given the diversity of religious beliefs, health-care practitioners should not seek to impose their own beliefs on patients, particularly when such beliefs conflict with generally accepted standards of medical treatment. In some instances religious beliefs extend as far as rejecting medical advice, as do the Christian Scientists. Nevertheless, rights carry responsibilities, and both patients and health-care practitioners have rights and responsibilities, enabling both to retain their autonomy within the limits of the law [see Exercises 2–9].

Guiding ethical conduct

The law is distinct from ethics. Law is used to emphasize and enforce those areas of ethical conduct that are agreed upon and defined. The law, however, can only act as a framework for settling differences in those areas of professional conduct where there is no consensus and in areas that are disputed but have not been resolved. There is therefore an interface between ethical conduct and the law that must be constantly borne in mind, even in emergency situations.

Urgent or emergency circumstances usually afford little time to resolve issues in the courts, and more and more institutions are turning to forums such as ethical committees to guide health-care practitioners in situations of conflict. This need is equally acute outside the institutional setting, and professional bodies should undertake the responsibility of providing guidance for their members who do not have an institutional base.

Ethical conduct in medical practice is by no means a new concern. The famous Hippocratic oath (see Figure 1) was formulated in the fifth century BC, and there were codes of conduct in ancient Egypt before that. Although the Hippocratic oath is still widely referred to as if it were a current code, an examination of Hippocrates' original text shows why society has to review its concepts of ethics and morality at intervals, for circumstances and thinking change. A review of ethical principles is particularly important given the religious pluralism that is enshrined in the constitutions and laws of many societies. In addition, the rapidity with which biological technologies change inevitably poses a challenge to previous moral precepts, for some of these technologies challenge the definition of life itself.

At times, society may try to circumvent moral and ethical issues and opt for what is often termed the pragmatic approach. For example, there is a widely held view that consent should not be necessary for HIV testing and that the results of such tests should not be kept confidential. These views are based on the fact that many other routine blood tests are carried out without explicit consent and on the belief that, because AIDS resulting from HIV infection is a transmissible fatal disease, those affected should be identified. Such "pragmatic" approaches often reflect a failure or inability to address all the relevant issues. There are many situations in which members of the public are unsure whether the right thing has been done to or for them, what their rights are, or what the obligations of health professionals should be in relation to their care. It is in these circumstances that sound ethical practice is particularly important.

At present there appears to be a strong public perception that health-care practice should be conducted within a better ethical framework, and some health-care professionals view this concern as fashionable or even political. The view also exists that this public perception has arisen because of a decline in religious adherence and a corresponding growth of faith in technology. Problems always occur when the foundations of faith are placed in doubt or shown to be false.

It appears that technology has become a religion for some medical professionals and laypersons as well. Practitioners and patients alike have been known to ignore accepted standards of ethical conduct in order to apply new technologies; in some cases, such as cloning, there may be a call to access new technologies without a full understanding of the ethical implications. Regardless of the widely proclaimed "miracles" of modern medicine, technology cannot and probably will never defeat all health problems. It is vital, therefore, that right and wrong practice within health care

Figure 1

The Hippocratic Oath

I swear by Apollo Physician and Aesculapius and Hygeia and Panacea and all the gods and goddesses, making them my witnesses, that I will fulfil according to my ability and judgment this oath and this covenant:

To hold him who has taught me this art as equal to my parents and to live my life in partnership with him, and if he is in need of money to give him a share of mine, and to regard his offspring as equal to my brothers in male lineage and to teach them this art – if they desire to learn it – without fee and covenant; to give a share of precepts and oral instruction and all the other learning to my sons and to the sons of him who has instructed me and to pupils who have signed the covenant and have taken an oath according to the medical law, but to no one else.

I will apply dietetic measures for the benefit of the sick according to my ability and judgment; I will keep them from harm and injustice.

I will neither give a deadly drug to anybody if asked for it, nor will I make a suggestion to this effect. Similarly, I will not give to a woman an abortive remedy. In purity and holiness I will guard my life and my art.

I will not use the knife, not even on sufferers from stone, but will withdraw in favour of such men as are engaged in this work.

Whatever houses I may visit, I will come for the benefit of the sick, remaining free of all intentional injustice, of all mischief and in particular of sexual relations with both female and male persons, be they free or slaves.

What I may see or hear in the course of the treatment or even outside of the treatment in regard to the life of men, which on no account must be spread abroad, I will keep to myself, holding such things shameful to be spoken about.

If I fulfil this oath and do not violate it, may it be granted to me to enjoy life and art, being honoured with fame among all men for all time to come; if I transgress it and swear falsely, may the opposite to all this be my lot.

be kept under constant review, not only within the traditional health-care professions but through the wider lens of social, legal and religious concerns.

Increasingly, health-care professionals must take into account that the public receives much of its information on medical problems through the popular media of television, newspapers, magazines and the Internet, and that most of the information accessed globally comes from the most litigious society on Earth. Because the United States dominates the mass media, the wider global public may expect conclusions and outcomes that are expected in the United States. Such expectations are inevitable if an examination of the issues is not undertaken within the social, cultural and economic context of their own societies.

There is danger in relying on the mass media or on any other public entity to determine a code of conduct for the health professions, for standards of practice and ethics differ markedly between the medical and other professions. It is not unusual to see tensions develop between the health-care system and other systems – most easily seen in the areas of advertising and disclosure [see Exercise 10].

In terms of health-care ethics, public attention has been focused on the doctor-patient relationship, human reproduction, genetic research, organ transplantation, AIDS, death and dying, access to health services, health financing and the allocation of health resources. How these are approached may have some universally defined parameters, but the conclusions each society reaches must be related to its own sociocultural and economic context [see Exercises 11–17].

In most countries the ethics of the health professions are imparted during undergraduate or other basic training programmes, and are expected to be monitored through the councils or boards governing the professions. The health professions' councils and boards are usually governed by the professions themselves and may be seen by members of the public to be self-serving. Thus, in spite of the complaints that are articulated privately (and sometimes publicly), the public seldom engages the professions through their councils and boards.

The public places the onus on the training institutions to produce the "right" persons, and the institutions may expect that much of what is taught will be reinforced by role models and the process of apprenticeship. However, if the role models have only absorbed the old teachings and precepts, without having examined the wider issues of today or assessed what is faulty in their own practice, it is not surprising that concern is expressed about the ethical conduct of today's health professionals.

The health professions cannot rely on the good old days, for they were not always so good. Two historical epidemics provide evidence: patients with cholera were abandoned and even ordered to be buried alive, and consumptives (people with tuberculosis) were described as "dissolute, dissipated and vicious" and locked away for the common good. This bit of history finds its modern parallel in the initial social and professional response to AIDS patients. When called upon to respect the rights of HIV and AIDS patients, many laypersons as well as health-care professionals asserted that rights were being invented for these patients that would endanger both the professionals who treated them and the general public. Professionals asked why they should not have the right to carry on as they had before, doing what they felt was best whether the patient liked it or not. This paternalistic approach to health care is under serious challenge, and ethical training must focus on helping health professionals adopt a more participatory approach that fully honours the autonomy of the patient.

Exercises 1 to 17

The following scenarios are based on events in practice. Identify the ethical and legal issues and state whether the conduct of the professionals was correct and why. If the professional conduct was not correct, state what it should have been. Discussion follows the exercises.

◆ Exercise 1

A 35-year-old married woman had complications during her fourth pregnancy, as a result of which her fourth child was stillborn. Her other three children are alive and well, although one of them has Down syndrome and requires special schooling. Her obstetrician has told her that another pregnancy is likely to have more serious complications and has advised her that she should be sterilized. She declined to be sterilized, telling her obstetrician that she did not want an operation. After discussion about possible complications, she was offered oral contraceptives. She accepted the prescription and made an appointment to see her general practitioner. Her general practitioner agrees with the obstetrician's opinion that it would be hazardous to have more children, talks about the dangers of oral contraceptives, and says she should consider the teachings of their church and use abstinence or the rhythm method. The consultation is concluded by the practitioner's asking her to talk to their priest about the matter.

◆ Exercise 2

A 15-year-old girl complains of nausea and vomiting and is sent to see her doctor, who asks about her menstrual periods and is told that they are normal. Finding no abnormality on abdominal examination, the doctor prescribes an anti-emetic and advises the girl to come back if the condition does not settle. The condition does not settle and she is taken by her mother to see another doctor, who tells the girl that he thinks she could be pregnant and will send a sample to the lab to confirm it. The girl begs the doctor not to tell her mother, refuses to take the test and asks the doctor if she can get rid of the baby. The doctor responds that he does not kill babies, even if the law allows it, and tells the girl that as far as he is concerned she has to have the baby.

◆ Exercise 3

A 42-year-old childless woman has undergone an *in vitro* fertilization procedure, and the pregnancy is proceeding with eight live foetuses. Her health has not been robust, and her doctors advise her and her husband that unless some of the foetuses are removed, in their opinion all the foetuses are threatened and the woman's life may also be in danger. After consulting their priest, the patient and her husband tell the doctors that they cannot agree to "killing" any of their "babies".

◆ Exercise 4

A woman has sustained multiple injuries in a motor vehicle accident. She is brought to the emergency department unconscious and in shock, with an obviously deformed leg from a broken femur. Resuscitation measures are started with the infusion of saline, and blood is sent for group and cross-match. It is determined that she is bleeding into her chest and abdomen. A chest tube is inserted and she is sent to the surgical department, where she is examined and it is noted that her blood pressure has improved to 100/80 and there are no localizing neurological signs. It is decided to take her directly to the operating theatre and obtain X-rays on the way to the theatre. As the patient reaches the operating theatre, a message is passed to the surgeon and the anaesthetist saying that the patient's mother has arrived at the hospital and has said that she is a Jehovah's Witness and her daughter is not to get any blood.

◆ Exercise 5

A Jewish couple with a family history of haemophilia on the mother's side has just had a male child. The mother wants the child circumcised by the rabbi, but the child's father insists that the circumcision should be done in hospital. The father takes the infant to see the doctor who deals with the family's haemophilia problems. The doctor examines the child and tells the father that the penis is normal and does not require circumcision, particularly with the child's demonstrated haemophilia. The father remarks to the doctor, "Surely it can be done safely if he gets plasma?"

◆ Exercise 6

A 55-year-old man is admitted to hospital complaining of lower abdominal pain, constipation and fever. He refuses to be examined by the doctor on duty, and when asked for an explanation he states that his religion does not allow him to be examined by a woman.

◆ Exercise 7

A 60-year-old woman who has been admitted to hospital makes it clear that she does not eat anything with beef in it and would prefer vegetarian meals. At each meal she makes a point of asking if there is any beef in the food. At one mealtime soup is sent up from the kitchen, and the nurse notices that it contains beef. She rings the kitchen and says to the dietary supervisor, "You know Mrs Singh does not eat beef; can you send up something else?" The supervisor responds, "Nothing else is prepared today, she will have to eat what else there is, unless you want to take the meat out of the soup; it would be vegetarian then." The nurse says, "I think that would still be against her religion." The supervisor responds, "I have a hard enough time cooking two pots a day; I can't deal with the ones who say they don't eat pork and beef."

Exercise 8

A middle-aged woman, found in a collapsed state in the street, is taken to hospital, where the diagnosis is made of diabetic coma and appropriate treatment is initiated. The only information known about her is from the workman who found her, who says she "probably works at the Christian Scientists' place". By the following morning she is improving . A woman calls the ward, identifies herself as the patient's employer and says that the patient has no contact with her relatives, and she knows that as a Christian Scientist the patient would not wish to be medicated. The physicians conclude that this information is almost certainly correct, given the way the patient was found. One of the doctors remarks that she will probably sue the hospital if she recovers.

Exercise 9

A 25-year-old Rastafarian woman is admitted to hospital with a three-day history of muscle pain and fever. She is delirious and dehydrated, and the doctor on duty makes a diagnosis of dengue fever complicated by the use of marijuana. The doctor orders that the patient's locks be shaved "for hygienic purposes" and informs the police that the patient has been admitted intoxicated with marijuana.

Exercise 10

A woman is referred to a surgeon with the diagnosis of gallstones. When she sees the surgeon she is accompanied by her husband, who asks the surgeon whether he uses the laser method. The surgeon says yes, and the husband asks how many procedures he has done. The surgeon responds, "You don't have to worry; all of the cases I have done have had none of the troubles you may have heard about."

Exercise 11

After several years of marriage, a 35-year-old woman has become pregnant for the first time. Her obstetrician has suggested that because of her age she should have an amniocentesis to see if the baby has Down syndrome. She asks what that means and is told that the child could be mentally retarded and might have other problems. She says she will have to discuss it with her husband, and an appointment is made for her husband to come in alone and discuss the matter with the obstetrician. During the discussion, the husband asks if other genetic disorders can be diagnosed at the same time. He is told yes but that additional tests are more expensive, and the doctor asks what it is that he is worried about. The husband replies that he would like to check whether he is really the baby's father.

◆ Exercise 12

A successful 60-year-old businessman has chronic renal failure and is on dialysis. His doctors have suggested that he get a kidney transplant and have asked whether he has any relatives who would be willing to give him a kidney. Several people make appointments to see the doctor to get tested, and the doctor realizes that they are not all relatives. One of the prospective donors asks the doctor if he can get some of the money before the operation.

◆ Exercise 13

A 25-year-old woman feels that she is pregnant and visits her doctor, who confirms the diagnosis, orders some blood tests and refers her to an obstetrician. A few days later the doctor's nurse calls to tell her that an appointment has also been made for her to see Dr Courtney. She asks why and is told that the doctor wants Dr Courtney to review her HIV test result. The next day the doctor gets an irate call from the patient's husband, threatening to sue.

◆ Exercise 14

A 65-year-old man with jaundice and itching is told he has carcinoma of the head of the pancreas. He consents to surgery and is told that if, at operation, cancer is confirmed and cannot be removed, a surgical procedure will be done to relieve the jaundice. After surgery his wife and children are told that he has had a palliative operation, and they ask the surgeon not to reveal the diagnosis to the patient since they do not think "he can take it". When the patient is awake, he asks the surgeon to tell him the full extent of the diagnosis and he is told that he had a blockage which was relieved.

◆ Exercise 15

A 92-year-old woman who lives alone is brought by her grandson to the accident and emergency department. During his weekly visit, he found that his grandmother was not her usual self: she had a cough and had taken to her bed. In the department she is examined, found to have an upper respiratory tract infection and referred for admission. The admitting doctor asks over the phone if the patient has any chest signs, and on being told no advises that the patient should be prescribed an antibiotic and given an outpatient appointment. When he is told that the patient lives alone and that her grandson works, the doctor responds, "I don't want my beds blocked by the elderly for care; refer her to the social services."

Exercise 16

A 95-year-old woman falls while going outside to bring in her laundry when rain was threatening. She sustains a hip fracture and is admitted to hospital, where she is entitled to "free" care. The surgeon advises that the fracture should be pinned, but the equipment is not available, and he further advises that she should be transferred to another facility to have the procedure done. The administrator responds that, were she younger, the hospital would be obliged to pick up the cost, but he thinks it best that she be left alone. The doctor agrees and orders that the patient be given anticoagulants for six months and kept in the hospital or sent home with 24-hour nursing assistance and daily physiotherapy visits.

Exercise 17

A 70-year-old retired woman who worked for many years in the local hospital has been under treatment for diabetes and hypertension and now has chronic renal failure. She is told that she cannot be dialysed since there are not enough machines, and dialysis is not offered to diabetic patients over the age of 60. When she protests, she is told to write or speak to the minister to ask that more funds be allocated for dialysis machines. She writes a letter stating that a person like herself, who has served so many years in the public service, deserves better treatment and that the money being allocated for treating AIDS patients should go to the dialysis unit.

Discussion

The following discussions address the issues of professional conduct raised in the exercises. Other conclusions are possible.

◆ Exercise 1

Issues

- Informed consent. Has the patient been given all of the information and the alternatives in relation to sterilization and contraception?
- The obstetrician's advice appears to be inconsistent with the patient's religious beliefs.

Professional conduct

- The obstetrician has given good technical advice but does not appear to have explored all of the avenues to achieve the therapeutic objective and has not taken into account the patient's religion or that of her husband.
- The general practitioner has properly explored additional avenues of contraception with the patient, but has allowed their shared religion to limit the alternatives that are given. The patient's husband has not been brought into the discussion.

Alternative approaches

- Both doctors should have asked the patient if she wished to include her husband in the discussion.
- Both doctors should have discussed a broader range of alternatives with the patient.
- The obstetrician should have considered the patient's religion as a pertinent part of the discussion and the advice given.

◆ Exercise 2

Issues

- Is the practice of the doctors within the normal standard of care?
- Parent's right to know. Should the doctor heed the girl's request that he not tell her mother?
- Is a doctor's refusal to treat within the law?

Professional conduct

- The first doctor falls below the normal standard of care in the history, examination and investigation necessary to come to a diagnosis. The second doctor meets the standard on the question of diagnosis but does not appear to obtain enough information to determine the best course to follow.
- If, as it appears, the girl has not reached the age of majority, the parents have a right to know about the child's condition under most circumstances. However, the doctor could accede to the girl's wish under the principle of the "liberated minor" if the doctor thought it was in the child's best interest to do so.
- A doctor has a right to refuse to carry out any treatment that he or she disagrees with, unless it is necessary to save the life of the patient in an emergency and there is no alternative. In this case, the doctor appears to go beyond the right to refuse to do an abortion and states that the patient will have to continue the pregnancy.

◈ *Exercise 3*

Issues

- Should a technique be practised that produces such an undesirable or dangerous result?
- Does a patient have the right to refuse life-saving treatment?
- Should the doctors seek to override the patient's decision?

Professional conduct

- Techniques in medicine are not as precise as one would wish. It is not unusual, in *in vitro* fertilization, for several foetuses to develop, nor is it always clear how best to deal with the situation. The doctors have acted professionally in giving their best advice to the patient.
- The patient has a right to refuse any treatment, even when it threatens his or her own life. Patients often wish to consult a clergyman in making life and death decisions.
- The doctors could at best try, by citing other opinions, to persuade the patient to change her mind.

Alternative approach

- The doctors could appeal to the court to try to compel the patient to follow their advice. This should be the avenue of last resort. In this case that approach would be unlikely to succeed, in the absence of a compelling reason to go against the patient's wishes and given the husband's acquiescence with her decision.

◆ Exercise 4

Issues

- Have the doctors acted appropriately in not obtaining consent to operate?
- Can the patient's mother determine what treatment the patient can have?
- If blood transfusion is part of the normal standard of treatment for a patient in these circumstances, should blood be given in spite of the mother's objections?

Professional conduct

- The doctors have acted within the normal standard of care for an emergency involving a patient who is unable to give informed consent. They have done an emergency surgical procedure without obtaining consent and propose to continue with the necessary treatment. Meanwhile, they should put in place mechanisms to find the patient's next of kin.
- The mother's status as the next of kin should be clarified by the doctors, since she refuses treatment for her daughter on the basis of her own personal religious belief. The patient's mother or father is the next of kin if the patient is a minor, and may be if the patient is an adult. A patient's spouse or adult children, if any, would supersede the parents as next of kin, and it would be vital to obtain their views.
- Refusal of a treatment measure by next of kin acting as a valid proxy must be respected, even though the measure is considered part of the normal standard of care in life-saving measures. Doctors may try to persuade the patient's proxy to reconsider but must continue to do all else that is possible for the patient.

Alternative approach

- A doctor who disagrees with a proxy's refusal to allow life-saving treatment can appeal to the court to be allowed to carry out the treatment.

◆ Exercise 5

Issues

- Should a doctor carry out procedures for religious purposes only?
- Should elective procedures not essential to life or health be carried out when the procedures are associated with significant risks?

Professional conduct

- The doctor has acted within the normal standard of care in the examination and investigation of the infant. However, the doctor appears to have taken little notice of the reason for the consultation, and the alternatives were not explored.

- A doctor does not have to carry out a procedure for religious purposes, particularly if it is considered dangerous to life or health. Normally there is little objection to circumcision of a male on the basis of injury to health. Circumcision of females is practised in some African cultures, but outside of those cultures it is considered injurious to health.

Exercise 6

Issues

- Has the patient the right to demand doctors of one sex or the other?
- Should the hospital administration acquiesce to the patient's request?

Professional conduct

- The doctor must respect the patient's right to refuse to be examined, and it is appropriate to ascertain the reason so that the problem can be addressed.
- The hospital administration should act depending on the hospital's rules regarding religious practice. The hospital may have a principle of respecting religious practices but may not have a staff structure that can satisfy this particular demand.

Exercise 7

Issues

- Should patients' dietary preferences be respected at all costs?
- What should the nurse do with what she has learned from the supervisor?

Professional conduct

- The nurse has conducted herself properly in monitoring the dietary preference and religious observance of the patient. However, she has not indicated what she will do about being told that other patients' religious dietary preferences are being violated.
- The dietary supervisor is aware of religious food restrictions, but does not appear to respect them if the patient can be fooled.

Alternative approach

- The nurse should report her conversation with the dietary supervisor to the nursing supervisor and ask for advice about how to deal with what she now knows about the food that may come up from the kitchen despite patients' expressed dietary preferences.

◆ Exercise 8

Issues

- What notice should doctors take of information they receive from a third party concerning patients' prior statements about treatment preferences?
- Should the doctors seek the patient's relatives and ask their consent to continued treatment?
- What actions should doctors take about the likelihood of being sued?

Professional conduct

- The doctors have acted properly in treating the patient in spite of the information they have received. They are acting on their own authority in an emergency, and there is no known alternative for treating the patient.
- In view of the perceived risk of being sued, the doctors should seek the consent of the administration to continue treatment on a patient who is unable to give consent and who has no known next of kin.

Alternative approach

- In the event that relatives turn up and refuse to consent to further treatment, the doctors should consult with legal and ethical authorities regarding whether the matter should be put before the court or if treatment should be withheld.

◆ Exercise 9

Issues

- Has the doctor diagnosed marijuana use on the basis of evidence or concluded it on the assumption that a Rastafarian must be using marijuana?
- Is shaving the patient's head justified for "hygienic" purposes, or has it been ordered for other reasons?
- Should the doctor report the use of an illegal substance to the police without the patient's knowledge or consent?

Professional conduct

- In the absence of a history or toxicology evidence, the diagnosis can only be described as speculative and should not be the basis for a report to the police.

- Without a specific statement of what the hygiene problem is, the doctor's order that the patient's head be shaved, knowing that wearing locks is a cultural expression, can be seen as an act of prejudice.
- The use of illegal substances should be reported to the police after the appropriate forensic evidence is obtained.

◆ Exercise 10

Issues

- Have the patient and her husband been fully informed about the proposed procedure?
- Should the surgeon have given truthful answers to the patient's questions?

Professional conduct

- The surgeon has not answered the patient's questions accurately: the patient may well be confused between the laser and the laparoscope, and the surgeon evades the question of how many of these procedures he has performed.
- The surgeon has sought to reassure the patient about possible complications and to avoid embarrassing the husband about his characterization of the procedure as being done by laser.

Alternative approaches

- The surgeon could have been accurate, without embarrassing the patient and her husband, by explaining the proposed procedure and the fact that circumstances may require that the "old fashioned" open procedure be done instead.
- The surgeon, in seeking to reassure the patient, should have been truthful about his or her experience and should have explained the precautions that would be taken to avoid complications.

◆ Exercise 11

Issues

- Has the obstetrician, after warning of the risk of an abnormal baby, adequately discussed the consequences of that possibility?
- Should the obstetrician have made the appointment to see the husband alone or should the consultation have been with the couple?
- Should the doctor have responded to new issues raised by the husband without consulting the patient?

Professional conduct

- The obstetrician has correctly brought to the patient's attention the risks of Down syndrome, but does not appear to have taken into account the special circumstances of the pregnancy or to have considered discussing the issues with the patient and her husband together.
- There does not appear to have been any discussion of alternatives if the foetus turns out to have Down syndrome.
- The obstetrician responds truthfully to the husband that a paternity test is possible and appears to agree to perform a test on the mother that has not been discussed with her.

Alternative approach

- The obstetrician should have seen the husband and wife together. If for some reason they could not be seen together, only the issues already discussed with the wife should have been discussed. If the husband did bring up additional issues, the correct response would be "We should discuss that together with your wife."

◆ Exercise 12

Issues

- Is the purchase of human organs legal?
- Is the doctor involved in this activity?

Professional conduct

- The purchase of human organs is illegal in most jurisdictions; however, the law is often silent on the matter. If the purchase of human organs is not legal, the doctor appears not to have adequately discussed the issues of organ procurement with the patient.
- The doctor, on realizing that a prospective donor was not a relative, should not have proceeded with the testing and should have discussed the matter with the patient before taking any further action.
- It appears that the prospective donor believes the doctor is involved in the purchase, and the doctor apparently does nothing to dispel that feeling.

Comment

- A surgeon has been struck off the register in the United Kingdom for being involved in the purchase of organs for patients.

◆ Exercise 13

Issues

- The doctor has ordered tests without telling the patient what they are, or obtaining her consent.
- Should the doctor or the nurse discuss this matter over the phone with the patient?
- Should the doctor refer a patient to another doctor without explicitly telling the patient the reason?
- What is the patient's husband suing about?

Professional conduct

- The doctor is treating HIV testing as a routine, non-threatening test, and has in essence committed a battery by not obtaining explicit consent to do the HIV test.
- The doctor appears to be avoiding responsibility for telling the patient about the result of the HIV test by referring her to another doctor and by asking the nurse to make the contact, and only when the patient questions it is there an admission that it is for "review" of the HIV test.
- In a matter as stigmatizing as HIV infection, the doctor is risking a breach of confidentiality by using the phone to discuss, even obliquely, the fact of an HIV test or a referral to a doctor who may be known in the community for dealing with HIV problems.
- On hearing from the husband, the doctor should be noncommittal and consult his legal advisors, giving them the facts thus far.

Alternative approaches

- The doctor should have discussed with the patient the need for an HIV test and obtained her explicit consent to the test.
- If an HIV test is positive, the doctor should ask the patient back without mentioning the test result. When the patient returns, the doctor should discuss the result of the test, including the possibility that the result could be a false-positive, counsel the patient and then decide with her what should be done.

Comment

- The patient's husband might be threatening to sue for battery committed on his wife. He may also feel that her confidentiality has been breached and that he is being slandered by the revelation of his wife's HIV status and the implications for his own HIV status.

◆ Exercise 14

Issues

- Should the patient have been told before confirmation of the diagnosis that he might have an inoperable cancer?
- Should the surgeon be speaking to the relatives about the outcome of surgery before the patient knows the outcome?
- Should the surgeon accede to the wishes of the relatives, against the specific request of the patient?

Professional conduct

- The patient has been properly informed about the diagnosis and the possibilities, yet when he asks for the full extent of the findings he is not given all of the facts.
- The surgeon is acting in good faith in trying to relieve the anxiety of the family but appears to have accommodated to the relatives' wishes without the consent of the patient, who appears to be fully competent.

Alternative approaches

- The surgeon should ascertain by inference or direct questioning how much the patient wants the relatives to be involved.
- The surgeon could explain to the relatives the importance of not deceiving the patient and arrange for the patient to have appropriate counselling and support when the true picture is revealed.

◆ Exercise 15

Issues

- Should the admitting doctor be assessing the patient over the phone?
- Is it appropriate to treat a person of this age and with this condition at home?
- Is the doctor discriminating against the patient because of her age and not discharging his duty to care for the patient?

Professional conduct

- The doctor in the accident and emergency department appears to have taken into account all of the circumstances related to the patient in advising referral.
- The admitting doctor has made no attempt to assess the patient himself or to ascertain by examination a critical piece of information that he or she is seeking.

- The admitting doctor properly has a responsibility to manage the beds under his care and to ensure that beds are available for those who need them. His remarks betray an attitude of discrimination against the elderly. However, a duty of care has been exercised, although the quality of that care may certainly be questioned.

Alternative approach

- The admitting doctor should have seen the patient and ascertained for himself any critical signs that would determine whether the patient should be admitted or not.

◆ Exercise 16

Issues

- Is the doctor consistent in his opinion about the best option for treatment, or does the opinion change based on costs?
- Should the hospital administrator be making decisions based on the age of the patient?
- Is the cost of the alternative care in fact less than that of the operation first proposed?

Professional conduct

- Presumably the doctor took into account the age and general condition of the patient in recommending the operation; therefore, his change of opinion does appear to be based on the costs as brought up by the administrator.
- The administrator quite rightly has to look at the costs of services; however, to use age as the apparent sole criterion is not appropriate.
- The doctor has proposed a non-surgical course of action, which should be costed to determine whether it or the surgical approach is justified. It may be that the full course of alternative treatment that the doctor proposed cannot realistically be carried out.

◆ Exercise 17

Issues

- Is the policy outlined fair?
- Should the doctor advise a patient to go to the minister for resources?
- Is the patient's approach a reasonable one?

Professional conduct

- Resources have to be allocated, and treatment may have to be rationed for one group or another. Such a decision should be scientifically defensible.
- It is appropriate to ask patients to advocate for themselves if other avenues have failed.
- It is unfortunate that the patient chose to approach the subject on the basis of earned privilege and by casting another group of patients as undeserving.

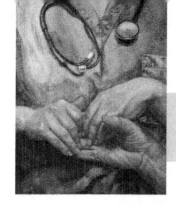

CHAPTER 2

Law and Ethics

While the law and its systems vary around the world, there are both commonalities and differences in ethical health-care practices. Concepts of ethical conduct in regard to specific issues may vary depending on where one practises. Medical practice has undergone more globalization than has law, and international organizations of medical and legal practitioners have forged codes of ethical practice that seek to establish an acceptable international code of ethical conduct in the practice of medicine; these include the Declaration of Geneva (Figure 2) and the International Code of Medical Ethics (Figure 3).

Most systems of law are structured to provide for different levels of adjudication, and there is usually provision for a final court of judgement where the law is interpreted and judgements are made in situations of uncertainty or where new situations arise. Ethical codes are guided by professional organizations that may be constituted at an institutional or state level. However, the enforcement of ethical conduct depends on the law of the land. It is therefore essential to understand the relationship between ethical conduct and the law in order to practise ethically.

The regulatory bodies responsible for monitoring and enforcing ethical conduct within the health professions vary with jurisdictions. There are also variants of health care–related statute law between countries, and, similarly, variations in state law occur within the federal structure of the United States. Health practitioners must be aware not only of the common principles that pertain to law in health care but also of the situations where local statutes vary. For example, the laws in the English-speaking Caribbean are derived from the English common law of the colonial period and therefore have similarities with the laws in England and in other British Commonwealth countries. With the exception of Guyana, the countries in the English-speaking

Figure 2

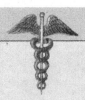

Declaration of Geneva (Oath of Professional Fidelity)

Adopted by the Second General Assembly of the World Medical Association (Geneva, September 1948) and amended by the 22nd World Medical Assembly (Sydney, August 1968) and the 35th World Medical Assembly (Venice, October 1983)

At the time of being admitted as a member of the medical profession:

I solemnly pledge myself to consecrate my life to the service of humanity;

I will give to my teachers the respect and gratitude which is their due;

I will practise my profession with conscience and dignity;

The health of my patient will be my first consideration;

I will respect the secrets which are confided in me, even after the patient has died;

I will maintain by all the means in my power, the honour and the noble traditions of the medical profession;

My colleagues will be my brothers;

I will not permit considerations of religion, nationality, race, party politics, or social standing to intervene between my duty and my patient;

I will maintain the utmost respect for human life from its beginning even under threat, and I will not use my medical knowledge contrary to the laws of humanity;

I make these promises solemnly, freely, and upon my honour.

Figure 3

International Code of Medical Ethics

Adopted by the Third General Assembly of the World Medical Association (London, October 1949) and amended by the 22nd World Medical Assembly (Sydney, August 1968) and the 35th World Medical Assembly (Venice, October 1983)

Duties of Physicians in General

A physician shall always maintain the highest standards of professional conduct.

A physician shall not permit motives of profit to influence the free and independent exercise of professional judgment on behalf of patients.

Figure 3 continues

Figure 3

Duties of Physicians in General (cont'd)

A physician shall, in all types of medical practice, be dedicated to providing competent medical service in full technical and moral independence, with compassion and respect for human dignity.

A physician shall deal honestly with patients and colleagues, and strive to expose those physicians deficient in character or competence, or who engage in fraud or deception.

The following practices are deemed to be unethical conduct:

  a) Self-advertising by physicians, unless permitted by the laws of the country and the code of ethics of the national medical association.

  b) Paying or receiving any fee or any consideration solely to procure the referral of a patient or for prescribing or referring a patient to any source.

A physician shall respect the rights of patients, of colleagues, and of other health professionals, and shall safeguard patient confidences.

A physician shall act only in the patient's interest when providing medical care which might have the effect of weakening the physical and mental condition of the patient.

A physician shall use great caution in divulging discoveries or new techniques or treatment through nonprofessional channels.

A physician shall certify only that which he has personally verified.

Duties of Physicians to the Sick

A physician shall always bear in mind the obligation of preserving human life.

A physician shall owe his patients complete loyalty and all the resources of his science. Whenever an examination or treatment is beyond the physician's capacity, he should summon another physician who has the necessary ability.

A physician shall preserve absolute confidentiality on all he knows about his patient, even after the patient has died.

A physician shall give emergency care as a humanitarian duty unless he is assured that others are willing and able to give such care.

Duties of Physicians to Each Other

A physician shall behave towards his colleagues as he would have them behave towards him.

A physician shall not entice patients from his colleagues.

A physician shall observe the principles of the "Declaration of Geneva" approved by the World Medical Association.

Caribbean have so far kept the British Privy Council as their final court of appeal to interpret their laws. There remain, however, some variations in law among these apparently similar countries: for instance, in Barbados and Guyana there are Termination of Pregnancy Acts which permit abortion under defined circumstances, whereas in other English-speaking Caribbean countries abortion remains illegal.

The professional conduct of health-care practitioners is regulated by laws that provide for councils or boards to examine the qualifications of the professionals; these councils or boards may administer disciplinary action for breaches of professional conduct. The composition and powers of the councils and boards vary from country to country, although the professional codes are similar. Obviously, practitioners should familiarize themselves with the professional codes of conduct where they practise. Practitioners who sit on these regulatory bodies must also be constantly mindful of their quasi-judicial status and conduct themselves accordingly [see Exercise 18].

Following is an example of what is contained in a professional code of conduct. Part V(2) of the regulations of the Medical Registration Act (1971–10), which governs professional conduct for doctors in Barbados, states:

> Professional misconduct includes any act or thing done by a medical practitioner that is contrary to the generally recognized duty and responsibility of a medical practitioner to his patient or that is contrary to medical ethics, or the failure to do any act or thing with respect to a patient in accordance with generally recognized medical ethics, and without limiting the generality of the foregoing includes:
>
> (a) adultery or other improper conduct or association with a patient;
> (b) any form of advertising, canvassing or promotion either directly or indirectly for the purpose of obtaining patients or promoting his own professional advantage;
> (c) wilful or deliberate betrayal of a professional confidence;
> (d) abandonment of a patient in danger without sufficient cause and without allowing the patient sufficient opportunity to retain the services of another practitioner;
> (e) knowingly giving a certificate with respect to birth, death, state of health, vaccination, or disinfection or with respect to any matter relating to life, health or accidents, which the medical practitioner knows or ought to know is untrue, misleading or otherwise improper;
> (f) the division with any person who is not a partner or assistant of any fees or profits resulting from consultations or other medical or surgical procedures without the patient's knowledge and consent;
> (g) the excessive ingestion of intoxicating liquor or drugs;
> (h) the impersonation of another medical practitioner;
> (i) association with unqualified or unregistered persons whereby such persons are enabled to practise medicine, dentistry or optometry;
> (j) the holding out directly or indirectly by a medical practitioner to the public that he is a specialist or is specially qualified in any particular branch of medicine

unless he has taken a special course in that branch and such special qualification has been registered in accordance with the act;

(k) commercialization of a secret remedy;

(l) knowingly practising medicine or treating a patient other than in the case of emergency while suffering from a mental or physical condition or while under the influence of alcohol or drugs to such an extent as to constitute a danger to the public or a patient; and

(m) the doing of or the failure to do any act or thing in connection with his professional practice, the doing of which or the failure to do which is in the opinion of the Council unprofessional or discreditable.

Thus, the law seeks to enforce some ethical principles, such as not having sexual relations with one's patients (a) [see Exercise 19]; maintaining confidentiality (c) [see Exercise 13]; exercising the duty of care (d) [see Exercise 15]; telling the truth, (e, h, j) [see Exercise 10]; seeking the patient's consent (f) [see Exercise 11]; and doing no harm (l, m) [see Exercise 13].

These ethical principles are universal, though not an exhaustive list as reflected in the international codes of conduct. The other principles in the legal code of professional conduct refer largely to relationships between practitioners rather than between practitioner and patients and are considered the code of conduct between professionals. Codes for professional interactions are more likely than those governing patient care to vary from country to country and between the health professions. For example, advertising is legal under US law but is still considered unprofessional by most professional associations in that country. In Barbados, advertising is stated to be unprofessional in the Medical Registration Act but is not listed as such in the Nurses and Midwives Act or in the Paramedical Professions Act, and many paramedical professionals take full advantage of that.

Each country has other laws that impinge upon the ethical and professional practice of health-care professionals. It is incumbent on health-care practitioners to know the laws that pertain to the profession in the jurisdiction in which they practise. There are also, however, some universal principles in law with which health-care practitioners should be familiar, including battery and negligence. Battery is a charge brought against an individual who causes harm to another by doing something without that person's consent. Negligence is a charge brought against a professional when harm has been done to a person by a procedure carried out without reference to the accepted standards of practice in the profession. A charge of manslaughter can be brought if there was gross negligence leading to death. As jurist Justice Lord Hewart put it, "The breach of professional duty has to be so great, that the negligence showed such disregard for the life and safety of others, as to amount to an offence against society and not just a matter of loss suffered by an individual patient" (Childs 1995) [see Exercises 20, 21].

In summary, ethical and legal codes pertaining to practices in health care are found not only in the laws governing individual jurisdictions but in international codes and conventions to which the individual country may be a signatory. These codes include the Geneva Conventions on Human Rights, the United Nations Convention on the Rights of the Child, Principles of Medical Ethics Relevant to the Protection of Prisoners against Torture and the codes relevant to the practice of physicians and nurses. The Code for Nurses is reproduced here (Figure 4).

Figure 4

Code for Nurses: Ethical Concepts Applied to Nursing

Adopted by the International Council for Nurses in May 1973

The fundamental responsibility of the nurse is fourfold: to promote health, to prevent illness, to restore health, and to alleviate suffering.

The need for nursing is universal. Inherent in nursing is respect for life, dignity, and the rights of man. It is unrestricted by considerations of nationality, race, creed, colour, age, sex, politics, or social status.

Nurses render health services to the individual, the family, and the community and coordinate their services with those of related groups.

Nurses and People

The nurse's primary responsibility is to those who require nursing care.

The nurse, in providing care, promotes an environment in which the values, customs, and spiritual values of the individual are respected.

The nurse holds in confidence personal information and uses judgement in sharing this information.

Nurses and Practice

The nurse carries personal responsibility for nursing practice and for maintaining competence by continual learning.

The nurse maintains the highest standards of nursing care possible within the reality of a specific situation.

The nurse uses judgement in relation to individual competence when accepting and delegating responsibilities.

The nurse when acting in a professional capacity should at all times maintain standards of personal conduct which reflect credit upon the profession.

Figure 4 continues

Figure 4

Nurses and Society

The nurse shares with other citizens the responsibility for initiating and supporting actions to meet the health and social needs of the public.

Nurses and Co-workers

The nurse sustains a cooperative relationship with co-workers in nursing and other fields.

The nurse takes appropriate action to safeguard the individual when his care is endangered by a co-worker or any other person.

Nurses and the Profession

The nurse plays the major role in determining and implementing desirable standards of nursing practice and nursing education.

The nurse is active in developing a core of professional knowledge.

The nurse, acting through the professional organization, participates in establishing and maintaining equitable social and economic working conditions in nursing.

Exercises 18 to 21

The following scenarios are based on events in practice. Identify the ethical and legal issues and state whether the conduct of the professionals was correct and why. If the professional conduct was not correct, state what it should have been. Discussion follows the exercises.

◆ Exercise 18

A 25-year-old woman notices a lump in her breast and goes to see her doctor, who is widely known as a breast surgeon, according to a sign outside the office. X-ray and ultrasound procedures are performed in the clinic, and she is advised that she needs an operation right away to remove a cancerous growth. The patient says she will have to discuss it with her husband. The husband says he is uncomfortable with the way his wife was rushed toward an operation and wants her to get a second opinion. The second doctor aspirates a cyst from the breast and reassures the patient that there is no cancer, and remarks that the first doctor does this all the time and is not really qualified as a surgeon. On hearing what has happened, the husband comments that he cannot understand how doctors can be allowed to practise surgery if they are not qualified.

◆ Exercise 19

A 25-year-old woman attends the emergency department after an accident and complains of pain in her shoulder. The doctor interviews her and asks her to go into the examination cubicle and undress. He performs a general examination, during which the patient feels that her nipples are being handled in a way intended to arouse her sexually. At the end of the examination she is told that she has no serious injury and that the doctor will call her the next day to make sure she is all right.

◆ Exercise 20

A 60-year-old man is admitted to hospital with a diagnosis of acute appendicitis and is taken to the operating theatre for appendicectomy. During the operation the anaesthetist remarks that the large swelling on the man's head made it a little difficult to intubate the patient. The surgeon says that he has never seen anything as large as that and he will take it out at the end of the appendicectomy. The patient makes an uneventful recovery but protests that the swelling on his head has been removed. A month later the surgeon receives a letter from the patient's lawyer, charging the surgeon with battery and demanding damages including loss of earnings.

◆ Exercise 21

A 60-year-old, very obese woman is admitted in a hyperglycaemic diabetic coma. She is treated for her hyperglycaemia and an associated bronchopneumonia. She is improving, but after a week confined to bed she suddenly has a cardiorespiratory arrest and dies. A post-mortem examination reveals that she died from a massive pulmonary embolus. Some months later the hospital receives a letter from a lawyer representing the relatives, requesting the notes on the patient taken during her admission. Several weeks after that a lawsuit is brought against the doctors, alleging negligence in failing to treat the patient to prevent pulmonary embolism.

Discussion

The following discussions address the issues of professional conduct raised in the exercises. Other conclusions are possible.

Exercise 18

Issues

- The first doctor appears to have made a diagnosis of cancer without confirmation on biopsy and is pressing the patient to have a surgical procedure performed on an urgent basis.
- The second doctor appears to have made a correct diagnosis, and makes a disparaging comment on the first doctor, placing doubt on that doctor's qualifications to practise.
- The patient's husband shows appropriate concern but does not appear to know what to do about his doubts about the first doctor's qualification to practise.

Professional conduct

- The first doctor is not acting within the expected standard of practice for the diagnosis of cancer, in that no attempt is made to confirm the diagnosis and the options do not appear to have been fully discussed with the patient.
- The second doctor acts within the expected standard of care; however, a doctor should not make critical remarks about a colleague to a patient.
- A doctor has a responsibility to report to the appropriate regulatory body if he or she knows that another "doctor" is unqualified to practise and is a danger to the public.

Exercise 19

Issues

- Is a general examination necessary, given the nature of the complaint?
- Can a patient distinguish between an examination and improper contact?
- Does the follow-up the doctor proposes give credence to the patient's suspicions?

Professional conduct

- There is a good rationale for the doctor to do a general examination; however, detailed examination of the breasts is probably unwarranted.

- The presence of a chaperone during the examination helps to avoid both improper advances by the doctor and incorrect inferences by the patient.
- Unless the procedure for follow-up is standard in the department, the doctor's proposal arouses suspicion.

◆ *Exercise 20*

Issues

- It appears that a large swelling on the head was noticed but not discussed with the patient.
- The surgeon may have thought it necessary to remove the swelling, after the remarks made by the anaesthetist.
- If recovery from the operation has been uneventful, how could a demand for loss of earnings be entertained?

Professional conduct

- If, as it appears, the swelling was noticed before operation, the surgeon or the anaesthetist could have mentioned it, which would have given the patient the opportunity to make known his attitude about its removal.
- The patient has had an operation performed without his consent, and this by definition is a battery. If it were necessary to remove the swelling as part of the procedure consented to or to ensure the safety of the patient, it would constitute a defence against the charge.

Comment

- It is possible that this man worked in a circus and made his living by being exhibited as an oddity.

◆ *Exercise 21*

Issues

- Should this patient have been treated to prevent deep vein thrombosis and pulmonary embolism?
- Can a suit of negligence succeed simply because the patient died of a complication?

Professional conduct

- This patient is classically at risk for the development of deep vein thrombosis and pulmonary embolism, and should have been treated with prophylactic measures.
- The case will be determined by the notes of the doctors and nurses. If prophylactic measures are recorded as having been carried out in a standard manner, the suit is unlikely to succeed.

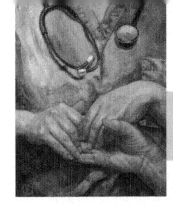

CHAPTER 3

The Rights of Patients and the Responsibilities of Health-Care Providers

W hen they find themselves enmeshed in the health-care system, people are at their most vulnerable, sometimes in fear of their lives, and they expect the health-care providers to help them through their illness and restore them to health. Responsibilities cannot be divorced from rights, and both are important to patients and health-care providers alike. Because patients are more vulnerable than the providers of care, their rights take precedence over those of the providers. Nonetheless, health-care professionals, who have the rights of any other citizen, also have special legal and professional privileges. This imbalance of power in the health-care setting means that health-care providers must exercise their responsibilities in a much more exacting manner than is expected of patients.

By law, health professionals are given the exclusive right to practise their profession without competition from unqualified persons. The legal right to exclusive practice is given by society to those who have the required training and qualifications, and is intended to ensure that the public receives a high standard of care. It follows that one of the health profession's responsibilities, which derives from the exclusive right to practise, is to ensure that high standards are maintained. Health professionals achieve this through keeping their knowledge up to date and through maintaining good professional conduct. The right to practise is not absolute, for the practice of medicine cannot be clearly defined or separated from home remedies, and "alternative medicine practitioners" can freely advertise, whereas in most jurisdictions medical practitioners are not permitted to do so.

Health-care professionals are given the right to determine the standards of practice in their profession and, within those commonly accepted standards, to prescribe, dispense and administer drugs and to carry out procedures that may be dangerous and can be associated with serious harm, including death. If an unqualified person were to administer similar treatment as a health professional and harm or death resulted, the person could be charged with a criminal offence, including murder. For the health professional to face criminal charges as a result of treatment, there would need to be a gross breach of the standard of care or a demonstrable intention to do harm. Although a civil tort of negligence may be brought against a doctor when a patient comes to harm, it can succeed only if the standard of care is shown to have deviated from the commonly accepted standard of practice in the profession. The extraordinary privilege given to health professionals in matters of life and death is given on the understanding that the professional will do no harm. Most societies therefore find it difficult to accept the idea of health professionals' deliberately causing death, even at the express wish of a patient – that is, euthanasia [see Exercises 21–23].

The professional's right to treat cannot be divorced from the rights of patients who come to be treated. In this regard the patient's right to know, understand and consent to being treated remains supreme. Even if the health professional considers a particular treatment vital, the patient has the right to refuse it. Any such refusal by a patient can be overridden only by the court. On the other hand, if a patient requests treatment that the health professional considers futile or incorrect, the professional has the right to refuse to administer the treatment. However, the professional should offer the patient other options and opinions [see Exercises 8, 11, 14].

Health professionals work in situations that may endanger their health, and they have the right to protect themselves from harm. However, choosing to be a health professional implies an acceptance of exposure to health risks, and the presence of such risks does not give the health-care worker the right not to treat patients. This became a highly contested issue with the advent of the AIDS epidemic, when many health professionals refused to treat patients who had or even were suspected of having AIDS. This behaviour illuminated the need, in protecting oneself, to first determine the risks, for adherence to universal precautions initiated to prevent transmission of infections to health-care workers was well within the scope of the training and resources available in most countries [see Exercise 24].

There are also rights and responsibilities connected to the handling of medications. A medical practitioner has the exclusive right to prescribe any medication that cannot be bought off the shelf. Nurses have the right to dispense and administer medications but not to prescribe them, except in some jurisdictions where certain categories of nurses have the legal right to prescribe a limited range of medications. Nurses, in administering medication, have the right and the duty to query any medication that they think may be incorrectly prescribed and to withhold the medication until the order has been clarified and confirmed by the doctor in charge. Pharmacists are not entitled to prescribe; however, they have the right and duty to query and clarify any prescription before dispensing it [see Exercise 25].

The following table summarizes the rights of patients and the concomitant responsibilities of health-care professionals.

Rights of patients	Responsibilities of health-care professionals
	Health-care professionals should:
Access to care Each person has the right to equal and timely access to health-care staff and facilities regardless of age, race, religion, gender, class, political or other affiliations. [See Exercise 15]	• facilitate access to care, particularly for poor, elderly and other disadvantaged persons • honour their duty to treat public patients in a timely fashion • refrain from exploiting public patients who seek timely access to care by asking them to pay for services
Respect for the individual Every person seeking health care has the right to be addressed with respect and dignity. [See Exercise 26]	• be sensitive to the feelings of patients and relatives and avoid denigrating labels for patients such as "social problem" and "elderly for care" • seek privacy for the patient even in the most challenging conditions
Religious and cultural expression Each person has a right to his or her cultural expression and religious practice and should be allowed to wear, use or have access to modes of dress and personal grooming, including symbols, provided that they are legal, not offensive to the rights of others, or breach the standards of hygiene and safety. [See Exercises 8, 9]	• avoid discriminatory actions – e.g., shaving a Rastafarian's locks without a medical reason • facilitate worship by the bedside where it is not possible for the patient to worship elsewhere, provided that the form of worship is not disturbing to other patients
Identification of staff Patients have the right to know the identity and roles of any health-care staff, including administrators, porters, etc., who are involved directly or indirectly in their care. [See Exercise 27]	• always identify themselves, even when they suspect that a complaint may be made *Table continues*

Rights of patients	Responsibilities of health-care professionals
	Health-care professionals should:
Confidentiality Each person has a legal right to privacy. Privacy includes information obtained from a patient whether it pertains to history, physical signs or investigations. It also includes the patient's diagnosis, treatment, outcome and methods of payment. Information should not be divulged outside professional settings, such as patient-care conferences and training situations. [See Exercise 13]	• keep all sensitive medical or social information within the health-care team • persuade patients, through information and counselling, to prevent the spread of infectious disease and in particular sexually transmitted diseases • warn a third party who is at mortal risk from a patient only after every effort has been made by and with the patient to avoid that risk, and only if the professional is sure that the third party is currently in danger • follow the direction of the court if ordered to break a patient's confidence • comply with the law regarding notification of diseases
Access to information All users of health-care facilities are entitled to information pertaining to the rules of the organization, including fees. Patients have the right of access to all information regarding their medical condition for the purpose of insurance or any other legal purpose and the right to obtain it in a timely manner. Patients are entitled to have the written opinion of the physician in charge in relation to the diagnosis, prognosis and advised course of treatment. Next of kin or guardians of the patient have the right of access to information in the same manner as the patient, only if the patient is not legally or medically competent to access the information themselves. Information can be given to relatives, including spouses and close relatives, only with the consent of the patient and in clear good faith if such consent has not been explicitly given. [See Exercise 28]	• try to ensure that patients receive financial and all other relevant information related to their care • provide certification for any legitimate purpose • provide access for patients to their medical information in a form the patient can understand • identify the legally competent relative/guardian to make decisions for minors and any adult who is unable to do so • keep up to date in their field of work so that patients can have the best advice *Table continues*

Rights of patients	Responsibilities of health-care professionals
	Health-care professionals should:
Other opinions Patients have the right of access to other opinions, medical or otherwise. The physician in charge should facilitate such access by making all relevant information available, providing it does not breach the ethical guidelines of the profession – e.g., referral to unqualified persons. [See Exercise 29]	• provide such information as the patient requires for access to other professional opinions • avoid referrals to or association with persons unqualified in the health professions
Consent to treatment Patients have the right to be informed about and to participate in decisions about their care. This includes examination, investigations and treatment of any sort. Explicit consent should be obtained for all procedures or investigations that may do harm, whether physical or mental. Patients have the right to refuse to be seen, questioned or examined in any way (including the perusal of notes) by anyone without giving explicit consent. [See Exercises 11, 20]	• explain all procedures, examinations and investigations, including their benefits and risks, in a manner that the patient can understand, so the patient can make an informed choice and consent to them • ensure that the patient understands any written form of consent and that there is no discrimination because of age in obtaining consent for treatment • counsel and obtain explicit consent for any blood test, such as that for HIV, the result of which may cause the patient to suffer from stigma in the community if the result were known
Refusal of treatment Any legally competent patient can refuse to be treated and must be informed of the medical consequences of the refusal. [See Exercises 4, 6, 8]	• respect the autonomy of the mentally competent patient or guardian to refuse treatment and ensure that their opinion regarding the treatment offered is clearly understood • continue to provide care and relief even in the face of a patient's refusal to comply with the treatment offered • facilitate access to second opinions and to senior staff

Table continues

Rights of patients	Responsibilities of health-care professionals
	Health-care professionals should:
Freedom from abandonment No patients should have their care abandoned unless clear arrangements have been put in place for their care to be taken over by a physician or competent health-care worker of their choice. [See Exercise 29]	• provide treatment for anyone coming under their care, irrespective of their ability to pay • treat any emergency to the level of their training and seek help where necessary • comply with the country's prevailing legal and ethical principles in matters such as euthanasia and withdrawal of treatment
Provision of basic necessities Patients are entitled to be provided with the basic necessities during their stay in hospital – including safe and clean surroundings and amenities such as bed linen and food. [See Exercise 30]	• request and be an advocate for the provision of clean and secure surroundings, adequate linen and nutrition as well as basic medical, nursing and other care
Security Patients have the right to be protected from physical, verbal and mental abuse by health professionals, relatives or visitors. Information on patients should be kept secure so that unauthorized persons cannot have access to their records. Patients have the right to bring before the authorities grievances and criticisms and to be protected from fear of reprisal, discrimination or limitation of access to health care as a consequence of any such complaint. [See Exercise 31]	• protect patients from harm which may arise from facilities, staff or visitors, including undue noise • ensure the safety of patients first in any emergency situation • ensure that patients are not being exploited financially, sexually or otherwise • keep records safe from intentional or accidental perusal by unauthorized persons • explain to patients, relatives and visitors how complaints should be directed

Exercises 22 to 31

The following scenarios are based on events in practice. Identify the ethical and legal issues and state whether the conduct of the professionals was correct and why. If the professional conduct was not correct, state what it should have been. Discussion follows the exercises.

◆ Exercise 22

Dr Kind is asked by the daughter of one of his patients to pay a home visit. The patient asks her daughter to leave her alone to talk to the doctor, who, on leaving about a half hour later, tells the daughter that her mother was very agitated so he has given her a sedative and she should not be disturbed for a few hours. Later that evening the daughter takes a supper tray in to her mother and finds that she is dead. She rings the doctor, who reassuringly says that this is how death happens at times. Dr Kind tells her that she could get the undertakers to remove the body, and he will furnish the death certificate. When the will is read, it is revealed that a substantial portion of the estate has been left to Dr Kind. The daughter contacts the police and says that she thinks that her mother was deliberately overdosed by the doctor.

◆ Exercise 23

A 45-year-old woman has a neurological disorder which has left her unable to walk without assistance. She drops utensils and is now unable to use cutlery to feed herself. She is unable to work, and her husband feels that his job is threatened as he has taken a lot of uncertified leave to take her for doctors' visits and physiotherapy appointments. On one of the visits to her doctor she asks if she could be given something that would put her to sleep so she would not wake up again.

◆ Exercise 24

An HIV-positive patient is admitted to the ward with a perianal abscess. This is drained routinely by the surgeon, who notes a papilloma on the buttocks but refuses the patient's request to remove it for fear that the site will become infected. When the patient's sepsis has resolved, he is booked for excision of the papilloma under local anaesthesia, and the surgeon is heard to remark that this is a good case for the intern. After the third cancellation, the patient complains to the surgeon that the intern keeps cancelling his surgery but is continuing to operate on other patients. When the surgeon asks the intern for an explanation, he is told that the patient's surgery was cancelled because he is too dangerous to operate on; the intern does not want to get AIDS.

◆ Exercise 25

An 85-year-old woman is admitted for colectomy for a neoplasm of the colon. Among the preparations for surgery, she is given low-dose heparin as prophylaxis against deep vein thrombosis (DVT). After the operation the patient bleeds unexpectedly and it is found that she has been given twice the dose of heparin prescribed. On enquiring why the patient was given twice the prescribed dose, the doctor hears a nurse remark, "The dose given was the correct one anyway."

◆ Exercise 26

A 90-year-old woman is brought for an appointment to a clinic and is taken into an examination room to be seen. Her grandson and other people who are waiting outside hear a loud voice saying, "Gran, you tell whoever bring you that they must bathe you before you come here next time."

◆ Exercise 27

A ward round is in progress. The group comes to an 80-year-old woman who was admitted the night before. The junior doctor says, "This is the old woman I spoke to you about last night. I would really like you to look at her belly; she doesn't seem to have settled." The senior doctor asks, "What's her name again?" After being told, she approaches the patient and says, "Mrs Peachtree, I just want to put a hand on your tummy," and pulls aside the bedclothes. The patient pulls the bedclothes back up and says to the doctor, "Nurse, the doctor examine me already this morning and I don't want any more prodding around, the belly hurting me bad enough already."

◆ Exercise 28

A woman rings Dr Garrett and says she would like a copy of her father's notes. Dr Garrett asks why, and she states that she is taking him to another doctor for a second opinion. Dr Garrett responds that he will prepare a summary but that she should bring a note from her father requesting the referral. The woman responds that she wants all the notes, not a summary.

◆ Exercise 29

A 72-year-old man has received a diagnosis of carcinoma of the bladder and has been advised by the surgeon to have an operation. He seeks a second opinion from another doctor, who explains that, depending on the stage of the cancer, it can be treated by surgery, radiotherapy or chemotherapy, or a combination of those, and that he should discuss these alternatives with his surgeon. When he consults the first surgeon, he is told that since he doubted his advice and went to another doctor he will not treat him anymore.

Exercise 30

A woman is visiting her mother in hospital and notices that the bed is wet. She asks the nurse if the sheets can be changed. The nurse responds, "Sheets are not changed during visiting time and in any case they have no clean linen on the ward. Why don't you bring in your own sheets?"

Exercise 31

A man is brought in to the accident and emergency department with gunshot wounds to the abdomen. While he is being assessed, two men try to enter the department, saying that they are friends of the patient and want to see him. The security guard tells them that the staff are attending to the patient and they cannot see him as yet. The guard thinks he recognizes one of the men as a former convict and asks the receptionist to call the police. On overhearing the guard's words, the two men leave the department; someone overhears one saying, "We'll get him on the ward." The incident causes consternation amongst the staff, and when the patient is due to be admitted to the ward, the staff protests, demanding that the patient be sent somewhere else.

Discussion

The following discussions address the issues of professional conduct raised in the exercises. Other conclusions are possible.

Exercise 22

Issues

- Is the patient's daughter justified in asking the police to investigate the circumstances of her mother's death?
- Should doctors accept such bequests from their patients?
- Has the doctor acted appropriately under the circumstances?

Professional conduct

- The doctor appears to have acted appropriately on the visit, although there was no report that the patient was agitated when the doctor was called.
- The doctor's reassurance is entirely appropriate, and although it is a sudden and unexpected death, the doctor saw the patient shortly before she died and could reasonably take the decision to sign the death certificate.
- If the doctor knows that there is a bequest for him in the patient's will, it would be prudent to ask the coroner to examine the circumstances of the sudden death after administration of medication and the request that the patient not be disturbed.

◆ *Exercise 23*

Issues

- Is this patient's condition terminal, and distressing enough to justify a request for euthanasia?
- How should the doctor respond to the patient's request to be put to death?

Professional conduct

- The patient's condition may be described as incurable, but not terminal. Her distress does not appear to be derived from physical discomfort but from her inability to help herself and the apparent downward economic spiral the family has been placed in by her illness.
- The doctor should pay attention to the patient's underlying psychological needs and economic circumstances, utilizing available social service and other referrals as appropriate.
- If the law of the land does not permit euthanasia, the doctor cannot lawfully entertain the patient's request. In the few jurisdictions where the law permits euthanasia, it is likely that there will be procedures to be followed to ensure that the patient's request is not a momentary whim, that there are no conflicting positions within the family, that second opinions are sought and that all available alternatives have been exhausted.

◆ *Exercise 24*

Issues

- Are surgeons who operate on HIV-positive patients placing themselves at significant risk of becoming infected with HIV?

- What is the appropriate response of the intern who has a fear of contracting HIV?

Professional conduct

- The surgeon has demonstrated that there are no extraordinary precautions required for handling an HIV-positive patient. The normal universal precautions of wearing gloves and avoiding injury while operating have been proven sufficient to prevent transmission of HIV.
- The less-knowledgeable intern apparently has an unwarranted fear and should discuss the matter with his or her supervisor rather than evading the issue to the patient's detriment.

◆ Exercise 25

Issues

- Does a nurse have any responsibility regarding the right dose of a drug?
- Can a nurse alter the dose of a prescribed drug without consulting the doctor?

Professional conduct

- The doctor has acted appropriately in providing prophylaxis for DVT and has used a lower dose than normal because of the patient's age.
- Nurses are responsible for knowing the usual dose of the drugs they administer and, in particular, for being cautious about administering too high a dose of a dangerous drug.
- When a nurse thinks that an incorrect drug or an incorrect dose of a drug has been prescribed, he or she has a responsibility to query the doctor about the prescription but not to alter the instructions, as appears to have happened in the case scenario.

◆ Exercise 26

Issues

- Does the staff show respect for the patient by not addressing her by name?
- Is the staff sensitive to the person's privacy, knowing their words can be overheard?

Professional conduct

- Addressing a patient by a title such as "Gran" may appear affectionate but may be taken by some patients as condescending. Unless health workers are truly familiar with the patient, they should use the patient's name.

- Any intimate statement to the patient should be made only after ensuring privacy. If privacy cannot be assured, then the point needs to be got across in another manner. Thus the staff member could have sought out the person who accompanied the patient and quietly told him the same thing.

Exercise 27

Issues

- Do the doctors act appropriately in their approach to the patient?
- Is there a good reason for the patient to mistake the doctor for a nurse and refuse to be examined?

Professional conduct

- The junior doctor shows a lack of respect for the patient by not addressing her by her name and referring to her as "the old woman".
- The senior doctor does ask for the patient's name. However, she has not been introduced to the patient by the junior doctor and does not introduce herself.
- It is not unusual for older people to assume that female health personnel are nurses, and the patient feels that she has already been attended to by the doctor.

Exercise 28

Issues

- Does a patient or a patient's guardian or surrogate have the right to obtain the patient's notes?
- Is the doctor correct in offering a summary only, and only after obtaining the patient's permission?
- Should all of the notes be supplied on request?

Professional conduct

- Information about a patient is the property of the patient, the doctor or the institution, where appropriate. The patient is therefore entitled to such information and can make the request through a guardian or legal representative.
- When requests come for information, it is appropriate to offer a summary and to ensure that it is the patient who is requesting the information. If there is any doubt as to the authenticity of the patient's request, the request should be put in writing by the patient or his legal representative.
- It is appropriate for all of the information to be requested; however, the doctor should retain the original notes unless ordered by the court to surrender them.

◆ Exercise 29

Issues

- When a patient wishes a second opinion, how should this be accomplished?
- Should the doctor giving a second opinion do so without the knowledge of the first?
- Is a doctor justified in not treating a patient because his or her opinion was questioned?

Professional conduct

- Patients seeking second opinions should attempt to obtain all of the information gathered so far; this may save unnecessary expense and will also make the first doctor aware that a second opinion is being sought.
- The doctor giving a second opinion should request from the patient all previous medical information so that the opinion can be provided expeditiously. However, the doctor is not obliged to notify the first doctor of the patient's request if the patient does not wish that to be done.
- The surgeon's response to the patient is unprofessional and is tantamount to abandonment of the patient.

◆ Exercise 30

Issues

- Why is the bed wet?
- Is the relative's request reasonable?
- Is the nurse's response appropriate?

Professional conduct

- The bed could be wet for a variety of reasons: the patient may have been sweating profusely, an intravenous infusion or drain may have leaked onto the bed or the patient may have urinated in the bed.
- The relative's request is reasonable, as she clearly discerns the patient's discomfort.
- The nurse's response is inappropriate in a number of ways. She displays no apparent concern about why the bed is wet or for the patient's discomfort or distress.
- The nurse, in seeking to explain the situation, has revealed a deficiency in the provision of basic necessities on the ward and has exhorted the relative to solve the problem, rather than suggesting that it is a problem for the hospital to correct.

◆ *Exercise 31*

Issues

- Did the security guard act appropriately?
- Is the response of the staff to the alleged threat reasonable?

Professional conduct

- The security guard responded appropriately to a request by either friends or relatives to see a patient who is being treated. The guard also acted appropriately on the suspicion that the "visitors" may have been criminals. However, it was imprudent to allow the suspected criminals to overhear the request that the police be called.
- The staff, while being properly concerned for their safety, should not seek to abandon the patient's care but should request additional security to ensure both their safety and that of the patient.

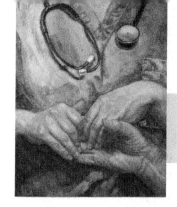

CHAPTER 4

The Rights of Health-Care Professionals

Professionals have all the rights of any other citizen as well as the exclusive right to practise their profession. In medicine the right to practise includes being able to prescribe medications and to carry out procedures that may cause harm or even death. Medical professionals' rights are limited and regulated by legal and professional codes which, when followed, make it clear that if some harm occurs during treatment it was not intentional. If harm occurs and can be shown to be due to neglect or to be intentional, then the professional is no longer specially protected and is liable under the law for negligence and even criminal charges.

When the rights of the professional clash with those of the patient, the rights of the patient prevail both ethically and legally. The issues that may place the rights of the professional in conflict with the rights or interests of the patient are confidentiality of the professional's medical information; the professional's right to practise his or her religion; and the professional's right to refuse to treat.

Confidentiality of medical information

A professional has the right to confidentiality of his or her personal medical information, as does any other patient. However, the professional and his or her medical practitioner have a duty to protect the professional's patients from contagious disease or any physical or mental condition that would compromise the care of patients and put them at unwarranted risk. A professional who has a contagious disease should not work during the period when the disease is transmissible. (Since most contagious diseases make the patient ill during the period of transmissibility, the requirement not to work seldom has to be enforced.)

Any dispute about the risk of transmission of a disease should be resolved on the basis of the available scientific evidence on the risk of transmission in the health-care setting. For example, it has been shown that hepatitis B can be readily transmitted to patients by health-care professionals in the workplace, but hepatitis C and HIV have been demonstrated to have been transmitted primarily from patients to health-care professionals. It is thought that, in one instance, HIV was transmitted from a dentist in the office. The evidence consisted of similarities in the virus infecting the dentist and five patients; however, no postulate was put forward to explain the mechanism of transmission (Ciesielski et al. 1992).

There is an effective vaccine against hepatitis B, and all health-care workers should, where possible, be immunized and should not be allowed to work until the viral antigen is shown to have cleared from the serum. Professionals infected with hepatitis C should not be allowed to work until the virus has been cleared from the body. As yet there is no certain way to clear HIV from the body; while HIV-positive health professionals can be allowed to continue working, they should voluntarily avoid doing invasive procedures where they are themselves at risk for injury.

In these situations the professional's medical information should remain confidential. This was upheld in the courts when the news media were prevented from publishing the HIV-positive status of two doctors in family practice. The grounds for the judgement were that there was no evidence that the doctors could transmit the virus in the professional setting. Therefore, there was no public interest that justified violating the confidentiality of their medical information [see Exercise 32].

Right to practise one's religion

Health-care professionals have the right to practise their religion but no right to impose their religion on their patients. For example, a Roman Catholic may exercise his or her right of conscientious objection to performing or participating in a therapeutic abortion. However, in those countries where abortion is legal, Catholic health professionals may declare their objection but have no right to put obstacles in the way of the patient seeking the service from another professional. In an emergency situation, it would be indefensible both ethically and legally to refuse to participate in an abortion without finding a competent professional to take care of the patient.

Jewish and Muslim health professionals should not advise circumcision on religious grounds to patients who are not of their faith. Jehovah's Witnesses may have a conscientious objection to the use of blood transfusion, but they would be ethically and legally wrong not to advise a patient about blood transfusion in situations where transfusion is considered the normal standard of care [see Exercise 33].

In countries ruled under Muslim law, a female health professional is not permitted to undertake the care of male patients. However, in other jurisdictions a female of Muslim faith will have a duty of care to both male and female patients [see Exercise 6].

A Seventh-Day Adventist and some Jews may claim that their faith does not allow them to work on their Sabbath. However, this practice cannot be justified either ethically or legally in health care, as the need for professional care cannot be excluded from those times determined by their faith. Any exercise of their faith that affected their work schedules would depend entirely on their eliciting the cooperation of others not of their faith [see Exercise 34].

Refusal to treat

A professional has the right not to treat a person by refusing a contract of service. There are several limitations on this right. Any professional who represents himself or herself as providing a service without stated limitations has tacitly agreed to provide the service to anyone who seeks that service. The contract of service is implied but can be refused if the person seeking the service has violated laws, such as threatening the professional, other staff or clients, or is unable to pay the previously stated fee for the service. These caveats do not apply in an emergency, where all professionals must render emergency care within the limits of their expertise and the facilities available [see Exercise 35].

Duty to treat in an emergency

The duty to treat a patient in an emergency is a matter of concern for some professionals, in that they fear being sued should something go wrong, particularly when seeking to assist persons at the roadside. The fear of being sued should be put in the context of the legal rights of the professional, for a lawsuit should not succeed simply because an outcome is not perfect. There are legal conditions that have to be satisfied.

Without a duty of care and in the absence of consent, a suit of battery could succeed. However, a professional who recognizes an emergency is committed to a duty of care within the limits of his or her training and the facilities available. The professional is also entitled to treat an emergency without consent if the patient is unable to give consent.

The results of treatment are often imperfect, but imperfection by itself is not a liability in law. To succeed in law the problem must be shown to have resulted from the treatment carried out and to have caused harm to the patient. Furthermore, if the treatment carried out was within the accepted standard of care for that professional in that situation, then the professional is not negligent by the standards established in law.

Therefore, the professional is protected from liability if it can be demonstrated that the treatment carried out was within the norms for the profession and for the area of expertise of the professional in question [see Exercise 36].

Exercises 32 to 36

The following scenarios are based on events in practice. Identify the ethical and legal issues and state whether the conduct of the professionals was correct and why. If the professional conduct was not correct, state what it should have been. Discussion follows the exercises.

◆ Exercise 32

The hospital administrator calls in Dr Bull and says, "There is a rumour going around that you have AIDS, and I am getting a lot of requests from patients to be transferred to other doctors, and the other doctors are protesting that they are getting all your work." Dr Bull responds, "I don't deal in rumours. If you're concerned, why do you not find out who is spreading the rumour?" The administrator says, "Wouldn't it be easier for everyone if you just got tested? Dr Test tells me that you've never had one done."

◆ Exercise 33

A 20-year-old woman is admitted to the ward for termination of a pregnancy. The doctor on call is called and asked to replace an intravenous line for the prostaglandin infusion being used to induce the termination. The doctor responds, "I am not coming to do it. The drip should be left down; we are here to save babies, not kill them."

◆ Exercise 34

A medical student about to take final examinations goes to the dean's office and requests that the examination schedule be changed because part of the examination falls on a Saturday, the student's Sabbath. The dean answers that the schedule cannot be changed for a number of reasons. The dean also remarks, "What have you been doing all these years, not attending Saturday classes or been on emergency duty? Surely you know that when you become a doctor you have to work on a Saturday?"

◆ Exercise 35

A journalist goes to a general practitioner's office and is seen by the receptionist, who fills out a patient record and takes it into the doctor. The doctor recognizes the name as that of a journalist who has written several articles critical of the profession, specifically about sick-leave certificates. The doctor asks the receptionist to tell the person that she cannot be seen today.

Exercise 36

A 20-year-old man fell off his motorcycle and is brought to the accident and emergency department, where an X-ray shows he has a fracture of the skull. He is admitted for observation. Three hours after his admission, the doctor on duty is called because the patient is complaining of a headache, feels drowsy and one pupil is reported to be larger than the other. The doctor asks if the patient has had a CT scan and is told no. The doctor orders a scan and asks for the neurosurgeon to be called. The response is that the CT scanner is not working and the neurosurgeon is not available. After the doctor sees the patient, who cannot be roused, the patient is taken to the operating theatre. In surgery, burr holes are bored and blood is let out. The patient's level of consciousness appears to improve, but four hours later he has a cardiorespiratory arrest and dies.

Discussion

The following discussions address the issues of professional conduct raised in the exercises. Other conclusions are possible.

Exercise 32

Issues

- Is the hospital administrator's approach appropriate?
- Is the doctor's response appropriate?
- Should the laboratory have given any information at all to the administrator?

Professional conduct

- Although the hospital administrator has a problem that needs to be addressed, the approach of repeating rumours is questionable. The administrator has also, quite unethically, obtained confidential medical information on a staff member.
- The staff member has correctly rebuffed any discussion of a rumour or of confidential medical information.
- The laboratory has acted unethically in giving the administrator any information on a staff member, whether positive or negative.

Exercise 33

Issues

- Is the termination of pregnancy legal? If so, is the doctor's response appropriate?
- Can the doctor's response be justified?

Professional conduct

- If the termination of pregnancy is being carried out within the provisions of the law, the doctor's response is inappropriate and amounts to neglect of the patient.
- The doctor could exercise a conscientious objection to participating in a termination of pregnancy, but where the procedure is legal the doctor should provide an alternative source of care rather than abandon the patient.
- The doctor has a right to his or her own beliefs but should not seek to impose them on the patient or on other doctors who are acting within the law.

◆ Exercise 34

Issues

- Is the student right in seeking to observe the religious day?
- How can religious-day observance mix with patients' needs for care on all days?

Professional conduct

- Everyone has the right to the observance of a religious day. However, health professionals cannot be absolved from the duty of care to patients, even on their religious day.
- The student may consider examinations and classes as not a part of patient care and almost certainly would have noted that no activities of that sort are scheduled for Sunday, a religious day for others.
- The dean's remarks appear to be insensitive to the student's religious observance and do not distinguish between patient care and other activities.

◆ Exercise 35

Issues

- Does the doctor have the right to refuse to see any person who comes to the office?
- Should doctors refuse to treat people who have been publicly critical of them?

Professional conduct

- A doctor, having offered a service to the general public, should see anyone who attends the office at the designated times.
- A professional should not discriminate on the grounds of race, politics, profession, point of view, or similar grounds.
- A professional may decline to be interviewed by a journalist if that is the purpose of the appointment.

◆ *Exercise 36*

Issues

- Has the patient been treated with the standard of care required in this circumstance?
- Should the surgery have been done by the doctor, who is not a neurosurgeon?

Professional conduct

- Although it would appear that a scan is the normal standard of care in this situation, there is enough information that the assessment could proceed without one. In fact, after the patient's condition deteriorates further, the doctor has to proceed without the scan.
- The narrative implies that the neurosurgeon should have been available but is not. Professionals should leave clear instructions of how they or their substitute may be reached.
- The doctor, despite not being an expert in the field, correctly deals with the emergency in what is judged to be a life-or-death situation. It is possible that the patient's life would actually have been saved by a neurosurgeon, but the doctor has done what appears to be within his or her level of expertise.

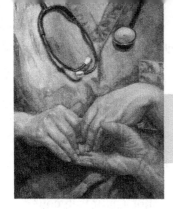

CHAPTER 5

The Duty of Care

ealth-care professionals, particularly doctors, are given the legal right to practise medicine. In practice, they may prescribe and administer medications and perform procedures that may have adverse effects. Provided the professional does not stray from the accepted standards within the profession, an adverse outcome is an acceptable risk. An adverse outcome resulting from the actions of a person who is not a professional is not protected; therefore the health-care professional has a unique right of care. The professional reciprocates this unique right by accepting the legal responsibility of a duty of care to any patient who asks for care [see Exercise 21].

The professional's training and the structure of the services offered often determine that a particular patient might be better dealt with by another professional. However, the professional should not refuse to see a patient until an alternative form of assistance has been found. This duty of care is clearly expressed in the regulations pertaining to professional conduct – for example, the Medical Registration Act (1971) in Barbados states that it is misconduct "to abandon a patient in danger without sufficient cause and without allowing the patient sufficient opportunity to retain the services of another practitioner". The duty to the patient is also addressed in a clause dealing with when the practitioner should not practise: "knowingly practising medicine or treating a patient except in an emergency while suffering from a mental or physical condition or while under the influence of alcohol or drugs to such an extent as to constitute a danger to the public or a patient" is also defined as misconduct. Therefore, even in the most adverse circumstances the duty of care should be exercised in the treatment of emergencies [see Exercises 36, 38].

The duty of care begins for the health professional when a "contract" has been made with the patient. A contract can be made orally and is implied when a service is offered to the public and a person accesses the service offered. An independent practitioner has a duty of care to all those who access the service he or she offers, and the employees of an institution have a duty of care to those persons who access the services offered by the institution [see Exercise 35].

Institutions are often organized so that the services offered are assigned to different categories of employees. The institution's rules should be known to the employees, and preferably published by the institution as rules of conduct. The client can break the contract for service by not adhering to the terms of the contract – for example, by not paying the fees, failing to obey the rules of the organization or engaging in criminal behaviour directed at employees or property. However, professionals must realize that their contractual obligation cannot be broken in an emergency medical situation or when a client's behaviour is due to a medical condition [see Exercise 38].

Many professionals express fears related to accepting the duty of care in association with roadside emergencies, violent criminals and HIV-infected people. Claims have been made against professionals who have acted in a "good Samaritan" role, suggesting that subsequent disabilities are the result of improper care. Such lawsuits can be defended as long as the professional has acted within the limits of his or her training and within the constraints of the circumstances. Professionals who find themselves in such situations should remember to record what they found and what they did and to pass that information on to those who take over the care of the patient [see Exercise 39].

Armed violence and criminals' pursuit of their victims into hospitals have led professionals to fear dealing with people injured in violent crimes. A professional has a duty of care to all patients, regardless of whether they are criminals. Such fears must be met by good institutional security, and while professionals must take all necessary precautions to prevent themselves from being harmed, the patient's safety and treatment must be assured first and foremost [see Exercise 31].

Many health professionals initially feared dealing with AIDS patients. A professional cannot abrogate the duty of care for fear of contagion or possible physical harm. The professional's training in universal precautions provides sufficient knowledge to protect against transmission of infectious diseases, some of which are far more easily transmitted than HIV. If professionals follow universal precautions, the risks of transmission of HIV in the health-care setting have proven to be minimal [see Exercise 24].

Exercises 37 to 39

The following scenarios are based on events in practice. Identify the ethical and legal issues and state whether the conduct of the professionals was correct and why. If the professional conduct was not correct, state what it should have been. Discussion follows the exercises.

◆ Exercise 37

Dr Night is off duty and has been at a party where he has had several drinks. After he gets home at 2:00 a.m., the phone rings, and Dr Sleep asks him to come to the hospital right away; Dr Cutright is having some difficulty with an emergency and needs a hand. Dr Night arrives in the operating theatre and scrubs, but in spite of all efforts the patient dies. On the way home he falls asleep at the wheel and his car runs off the road.

◆ Exercise 38

A 25-year-old man involved in a traffic accident has been admitted to the ward, restless and suspected of having intra-abdominal injuries. Dr Touchie is trying to put up an intravenous infusion on the patient, when the patient violently pulls away his arm and the doctor is struck in the face. Dr Touchie declares, "I am having nothing more to do with this man," and leaves the ward.

◆ Exercise 39

Dr Samar is driving home when an accident occurs up ahead of him. He noticed that two cars were racing, and one got out of control and slammed into another car going in the opposite direction. Dr Samar pulls over and sees that the driver of one of the cars is trapped behind the wheel with his seat belt on, and the other driver is walking away from his car. Dr Samar introduces himself, helps the driver out of the car and asks the driver how he feels. The driver responds, "A little shaken but all right." Dr Samar says, "Let me look at your chest." He notices the mark made by the seat belt and says, "You are lucky; it looks like the seat belt saved you, but you better get yourself checked out." The ambulance arrives on the scene, and Dr Samar leaves. The ambulance attendant speaks to the driver of the vehicle, who says, "Don't worry about me; Dr Samar says the seat belt saved me."

Discussion

The following discussions address the issues of professional conduct raised in the exercises. Other conclusions are possible.

Exercise 37

Issues

- Should the doctor, knowing that he has been drinking, respond to the call for help?
- Is the doctor liable if a lawsuit is brought alleging negligence for operating while intoxicated?

Professional conduct

- A doctor, even when off duty, may be called to deal with an emergency situation, and therefore should avoid becoming intoxicated.
- If a doctor is called on for help and feels unfit to help, he or she should say so. However, if there is no one else available and the situation is a life-threatening emergency, the doctor should assist to the best of his or her ability.
- If a doctor responds to an emergency situation while intoxicated and there were no other alternatives available, the action could be defended on the basis of duty of care in an emergency.

Exercise 38

Issues

- Is the doctor justified in abandoning the patient?
- How should this patient be dealt with?

Professional conduct

- The patient may be violent for a number of reasons: he may be going into shock, may be hypoxic, may be intoxicated or may be resisting the attempted procedure.
- The doctor cannot justifiably leave the patient, who may be in danger, without providing alternative care. The patient may be sedated with the help of others and treated appropriately.

◆ *Exercise 39*

Issues

- Has the doctor acted properly in response to the accident?
- Is the driver correct to be reassured with the doctor's opinion?

Professional conduct

- The doctor has acted properly as a good Samaritan and stopped at the scene of the accident. In looking at the trapped driver, he has correctly identified himself as a doctor and presumably has judged that it is safe to move the driver.
- In assessing the injury, the doctor has done what he can do at the roadside. Although he makes a reassuring remark, he also advises the patient to seek further assessment. Unfortunately, the patient appears to have taken the doctor's reassurance but not the caution.
- The doctor, having in essence assessed the patient, should not have left the scene without telling the ambulance personnel both his assessment and his advice for follow-up.

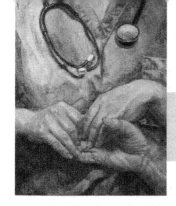

CHAPTER 6

Confidentiality

Confidentiality is a cornerstone of the relationship between the patient and the health professional. That relationship is based on the patient's trust that sensitive personal information or findings will remain within the professional setting. Without that trust patients will not seek advice, may withhold information important to the diagnosis of their condition and may not accept therapeutic advice for fear that they will be embarrassed by disclosure to others. The principle of confidentiality not only is enshrined in the ethical codes but also is a fundamental right in law [see Exercise 40].

The law

In many countries, the right to confidentiality is expressed as a constitutional right to privacy. The right to privacy is also found in the International Convention on Human Rights, to which most countries are signatories. Confidentiality is specifically protected in the laws governing the conduct of the health professions; for example, in Barbados the Regulations for the Medical Registration Act (1971) state that the "wilful or deliberate betrayal of a professional confidence" constitutes an offence, and similar provisions are found in the Dental, Nurses and Midwives, and Paramedical Professions Registration Acts. However, these laws do not necessarily provide sufficient protection for the patient with respect to national and other insurance agencies and the linking of medical records to other identifiers such as national registration numbers. Some countries have passed specific acts to safeguard the confidentiality of information while allowing patient information to be used for regulatory and research purposes.

The law also contains specific exceptions which address matters related to public health regulations and criminal proceedings. It is therefore incumbent on health-care workers to be familiar with the specific acts in the jurisdiction where they practise. For example, confidentiality has to be broken to accommodate the provision of information for notifiable diseases, but the list of notifiable diseases varies from country to country. Most notably, sexually transmitted diseases are not notifiable diseases in all countries. This has proven to be of major importance in dealing with the stigmatizing condition of HIV/AIDS, for many patients would be understandably reluctant to be tested for HIV if they believed their status would become known to the public. Similarly, doctors are often reluctant to comply with the law governing notification if their patient's confidentiality cannot be assured. Although patients seldom seek legal sanctions for a breach of confidentiality by itself, a breach usually sets the stage for disgruntled patients to look for, or join to a breach of confidentiality, other wrongs which they feel they might have suffered.

The health-care team

Although confidentiality applies to all information related to a patient's medical condition and treatment, it is not synonymous with secrecy, for modern treatment requires the flow of information among professionals. Breaching of confidentiality occurs when information is divulged to unauthorized third parties who use it to the patient's disadvantage. Many people are involved in the modern health-care system, and while health-care professionals have regulations that govern confidentiality, there are other employees who do not; these employees should be bound to the principle of confidentiality by their employer in their contractual obligations. The doctor in charge or the employer can be ethically and legally liable for any damages that arise out of a breach of confidentiality by an employee.

Medical records

To protect the confidentiality of patient information, specific precautions should be taken with patient records, particularly those stored or transmitted in an electronic format. Thus, confidential information should be transmitted by fax only if the receiving doctor is available at the time of transmission, and e-mail should be used for the transmission of records only with the permission of the patient or with agreed security by encryption.

In general, patients have a right to their records, and when they request them they should do so in writing, even when it is their attorney who wants the records. This right to one's own records extends till after death and is vested in the executor or estate or, failing that, in the next of kin. In some countries there are limitations placed on the information patients can receive from their records – for instance, information contained in patient records that may refer to persons other than medical personnel involved in their care has been cited as a specific exception in the Access to Medical Reports Act (1988) in the United Kingdom. It is also prudent to consider whether information that could worsen the patient's mental or physical state should be revealed to the patient. Such considerations must be balanced against the possibility of being accused of withholding information for the benefit of the practitioner rather than the patient, and it is a good idea to seek advice in such cases [see Exercise 41].

The right to know

Who has the legal right to know anything about a patient? The answer is that only the patient or the patient's legal guardian and the doctor to whom the patient's care has been entrusted are entitled to confidential information. Where the patient's care has been entrusted to an institution rather than a specific practitioner, the institution also has the right to the information. It should be stressed, however, that occupational physicians employed by companies to look after employees have a primary professional responsibility of confidentiality to the patients they see. Any report to an employer, such as a determination of fitness to work, must be given only with the employee's informed consent. There are exceptions to these general provisions as required by law, and these are dealt with under the heading "Exceptions" below [see Exercise 42].

It is in the best interest of patient care that all professionals involved in the care of a patient should know all of the pertinent information about the patient. However, they do not have a legal right to this information. The best way for professionals to ensure that patient information is not withheld is to assure the patient and the doctor in charge that confidentiality will be maintained and that information will not be used to the disadvantage of the patient.

Within the family

Confidentiality can be a sensitive issue among family members in some circumstances; for example, contact tracing of sexually transmitted diseases (STDs) is usually sensitive since the sexual partner(s) may be outside the family. Similarly, disclosure of abortions or miscarriages may cause problems within a family.

There are occasions when patients do not wish family members to be aware of a serious and possibly fatal illness while they make arrangements for the disposal of their estate. Practitioners should never assume that relatives should know of a serious illness and should assure themselves that disclosure to family members accords with the patient's wishes [see Exercise 43].

In the workplace

In the workplace, fear of contagious disease and mental illness are common, and there are often strident demands that confidentiality about an employee's illness should be broken. Certification of fitness to work is the province of the medical practitioner only, and there is no duty or obligation to disclose a person's specific illness to the person's employer or workmates [see Exercise 44].

Insurance providers

Insurance agencies, including compulsory government insurers, demand diagnoses before they disburse benefits. Many patients, in spite of signing insurance claim forms revealing their diagnosis, feel that their confidentiality is being broken to persons who are not health-care professionals and who are under no obligation to respect their confidentiality.

An unfortunate custom has grown up of using a copy of the insurance certificate as a convenient certificate for the employer, and some employers have come to believe that it is their right to know the worker's diagnosis. The employer has no right to know an employee's diagnosis without the employee's consent. This applies even in cases where the employer is paying for the medical attention the employee is receiving [see Exercise 45].

VIPs

It is widely perceived that there is a double standard whereby great efforts are made to ensure confidentiality for some influential people, whereas little effort is made for others. VIPs, on becoming ill with sensitive diseases, often wish to forgo the publicity that usually attends their activities and wish to become another kind of VIP: *very intensely private*. In spite of any perception of hypocrisy, all people must be accorded equal rights to confidentiality, and press enquiries should be answered only with the patient's consent [see Exercise 46].

After death

The right to confidentiality does not cease with a patient's death, for a person's estate retains his or her legal rights after death. The rights retained after death include the right to sue for negligence – which contradicts the saying "Doctors can bury their mistakes." It is therefore possible that a civil suit alleging a breach of confidence can be brought after the death of the patient. It is also conceivable that relatives may sue over revealing the presence of an inheritable disorder, particularly if it carries a serious stigma in the community. However, the issuance of an accurate death certificate is protected in law, and scientifically accurate death certificates must always be issued [see Exercise 47].

HIV/AIDS

Because of the stigma and fear attached to AIDS and infection with HIV, both the public and health professionals have expressed concerns about maintaining confidentiality for those who are affected. Issues of confidentiality have been raised in relation to job screening, travel and immigration, transmission in health-care settings, surveillance and contact tracing. In many of these areas there have been deliberate attempts to breach confidentiality, either directly or by inference, to or by third parties.

With the exception of sex workers, there is no scientific rationale for HIV screening of workers. Screening of workers fosters discrimination and unwarranted actions, billed as precautions, in the workplace. Some employers have used the rationale of providing health-insurance coverage as the basis for screening job applicants. This approach implies that workers who have any of the screened-for conditions – such as HIV infection, diabetes or hypertension – will not have access to health care through private insurance agencies. Similar arguments related to the expenses of medical care are used to exclude HIV-infected persons and to justify testing applicants for immigration and even for travel in some countries [see Exercise 48].

Health-care workers have tried to justify HIV screening of patients on the grounds of protecting themselves. This cannot be justified scientifically or ethically, and where practised it has rebounded on the professionals. In the wake of a reported case of transmission of HIV in a dental practice, some members of the public have demanded screening of health-care workers, with a similar lack of scientific justification. In the United Kingdom the health department has ordered the screening of all new entrants to the National Health Service in disciplines that perform invasive procedures. No rationale has been given for the order, and there is no policy to exclude persons who are already in those disciplines who are HIV-positive [see Exercise 49].

As for surveillance and contact tracing, history has shown that with sensitive social diseases, maintenance of confidentiality is essential to achieving the aim of not spreading the disease, in contrast to what many people think. People who do not expect confidentiality to be maintained do not come for diagnosis early; they therefore may spread a virus like HIV more than they would have if they had sought a diagnosis knowing they would not face disgrace or discrimination through unwarranted disclosure.

Exceptions

Under certain circumstances, confidentiality can legally be broken without the patient's consent. These circumstances are described below.

Certification of death

Accurate certification of death is an essential surveillance tool for monitoring the health of the community. Correct certification should always be given, regardless of any social or other pressure to do otherwise [see Exercise 50].

Notifiable diseases

These are diseases, primarily communicable diseases, that the doctor is legally bound to report to the health authorities. Such notification is accompanied by information about the patient, such as name, address and occupation. The list of diseases varies depending on the jurisdiction. Notification is an essential tool in public health surveillance and the means by which authorities can act to safeguard the health of the community as a whole. There are sanctions for doctors who do not comply; however, they are seldom exercised.

The courts

A judge can order a doctor to reveal information about a patient against the patient's wishes. Normally such orders are exercised only when the information is pertinent to criminal proceedings. Most patient information revealed in court is done with the patient's consent in cases of injuries, accidents or proceedings related to a suit of negligence.

Third parties at risk

It has been established that a doctor can reveal patient information to a third party at risk from a patient, if certain conditions have been met. First, the risk must be a mortal one; second, the patient must know of the risk; and, finally, the doctor must know that the patient is putting the third party at risk without informing the person at risk. This provision arose in response to violent behaviour by psychotic patients in the United States [*Tarsakoff v. Regents of the University of California* (1976)]. It is widely debated in the context of HIV infection, with respect to both sexual relationships and needle sharing among intravenous drug abusers [see Exercise 51].

Minors

Generally, parents and legal guardians have the legal right to know all matters pertaining to the diagnosis and treatment of a minor. In most jurisdictions a person is a minor until the age of 18 years, although in some places the age of majority is 21 years, and in a few jurisdictions the age of consent may be less than 18 years. On a sensitive matter such as the use of contraceptives or an unintentional pregnancy, a minor may wish to take action (and the doctor may judge that action to be in the minor's best interest), but the minor does not wish her parent(s) to know. The situation may be complicated by the fact that a person younger than the age of majority – for instance, a 16-year-old in Barbados – can legally consent to intercourse but cannot legally consent to treatment for any of its consequences. As a result, some jurisdictions have established the concept of the liberated or emancipated minor – that is, a minor who has become a parent, or who can make certain decisions about his or her own care without reference to parents or guardians [see Exercise 2].

There may also be some specific provisions in the law related to minors. For example, in Barbados, where the age of majority is 18 years, the Termination of Pregnancy Act allows a 16-year-old to consent to the termination of an early pregnancy without reference to her parents. In the United Kingdom the Family Law Reform Act makes provision for a 16-year-old to act as an adult in consenting to medical care without reference to parents.

Infectious disease

Every person has the right to be protected from contracting an infectious disease. Provisions to breach confidentiality to protect others from contagious disease are usually contained in a country's public health regulations [see Exercise 51].

Crime

A patient may want personal information that pertains to a criminal act to be kept confidential. This desire may conflict with a health professional's ethical or legal duty to report felonies to the police. In those circumstances, the patient should be told that the practitioner has a duty to report a felony to the police; should the patient object to disclosure, the practitioner should seek legal guidance before making any disclosure [see Exercise 51].

Exercises 40 to 51

The following scenarios are based on events in practice. Identify the ethical and legal issues and state whether the conduct of the professionals was correct and why. If the professional conduct was not correct, state what it should have been. Discussion follows the exercises.

◈ Exercise 40

An operating theatre nurse notices that her husband has not been sleeping well and has been drinking heavily. She says to one of her colleagues, "You know, he keeps joking that there's an old story that if you give blood to anyone who dies that you will die next, and I know he went to donate blood recently for one of his drinking buddies." Her colleague says, "Sounds like you better find out what his tests showed." The nurse then rings the laboratory, identifies herself and asks if she could have the results of the tests on her husband's blood. After asking her to hold on for a moment, the lab technician gives her the results.

◈ Exercise 41

The hospital records department sends out a notice stating that from now on patients' records will be stored in the computer files and the national identity number must be filled in on all records. Dr Stickler writes and asks how the confidentiality of the patients' medical information will be protected under this new system. The hospital administrator sends out a notice stating that the government has decided to locate all records under a single number to improve the efficiency of transactions between departments.

◈ Exercise 42

A 17-year-old boy is seen in the emergency department complaining of fever, burning on micturition and discharge from the penis. The doctor diagnoses gonorrhoea, counsels the boy about safer sexual activity and suggests that he should take an HIV test. The boy says he would just like to be treated for the gonorrhoea and asks the doctor not to tell his mother, who is waiting outside.

◈ Exercise 43

Mr Peck consults his doctor complaining of abdominal pain and weight loss. He is accompanied by Mrs Peck, who answers all of the doctor's questions about the complaint and wants to stay in the examination room when Mr Peck is being examined. The doctor requests that she stay out of the examination room and asks Mr Peck if there is anything else about his symptoms he would like to tell him. Mr Peck replies that if he has a cancer he does not want his wife told because there is some business he wants to organize before she knows.

◆ Exercise 44

A 30-year-old man who has been having treatment for a lymphoma returns to work as a waiter at the end of two months' sick leave. His employer says he has a substitute working for the rest of the week already and asks him to request more leave from his doctor while the employer sorts out the situation. The employer rings the man's doctor and says, "Dr Doorite, I know that I shouldn't call you like this, but Ralph Table works with me and I notice you were treating him for a lymphoma, and there are rumours going around that he has AIDS. I can't afford to have someone with AIDS working in a business like mine, and I wonder whether when you write his next certificate if you could state that he will not be fit to wait at table. By the way, did you get those vouchers we sent you?"

◆ Exercise 45

Ms Pritty has applied for a mortgage at the bank and is told that they need to take out an insurance policy on her life to cover the mortgage. She is asked to sign the insurance application form and to take it to Dr Surance, who does the insurance examinations for the company. Some weeks after the examination, she enquires at the bank when she can expect the mortgage to come through. The bank officer tells her that they have stopped processing the application since her insurance was refused. She asks why the insurance was refused, and the bank officer says, "They didn't tell you that you tested positive?"

◆ Exercise 46

The Right Honourable Mr Wheel is admitted to the hospital. Dr Barrow gets a call from a member of the press, who says, "I understand from Mr Wheel's daughter that you are looking after him and that he is in for control of his diabetes. Can you tell us why his diabetes went out of control and how long he is expected to be in the hospital?"

◆ Exercise 47

An announcement is made of the sudden death of Mrs Eve, the wife of the prime minister. A rumour has spread that there was a domestic dispute and she fell down the stairs. Mrs Adam, her daughter, has spoken to the press, saying that Dr Hart has been attending her mother for 20 years and has confirmed that she died from a heart attack. Dr Hart is called by a journalist and asked if he will confirm what was said by Mrs Adam and if a post-mortem will be done.

◆ Exercise 48

The government has announced its policy on the control of HIV. It states that, in keeping with the government's respect for human rights, there should be no screening of job applicants for HIV. This policy is justified on the grounds that HIV is not transmitted in the workplace and that being HIV-positive is a chronic condition with which people can be well and productive for many years, rather than being a charge on the community and the government through being unable to find work. Someone calls a call-in programme and asks if this means that the government will now stop screening its own job applicants. The ministry's public relations officer calls in to deny that government departments have a screening policy, and states that any testing that is done is for the health insurance that all employees are entitled to. Dr Too, who has been screening job applicants for the government, writes the ministry to ask for a clarification of its policy.

◆ Exercise 49

Dr Safer is well known around the hospital for insisting that HIV testing be done on all patients on whom he is doing a major operation. One evening he is brought into the accident and emergency department after being involved in a motor vehicle accident. He is suspected of having intra-abdominal bleeding, and the surgeon on duty is called. The surgeon asks whether an HIV test has been done. The officer on duty tells Dr Safer that the surgeon has asked for an HIV test and Dr Safer shouts, "I don't want that idiot touching me, get someone else!"

◆ Exercise 50

Dr Easer is called to the home of a patient of his who has taken an overdose of pills. The patient is admitted to the hospital, the pills are pumped out of the stomach and measures are taken to counteract the effect of the drugs. In spite of these measures, the patient develops liver failure and dies while awaiting liver transplantation. Dr Easer rings the mother of the patient to inform her of her daughter's death. She asks him what he will put on the death certificate: "Please do not put down suicide."

◆ Exercise 51

Dr Dolema is seeing Mr Bisic for a recurrence of genital herpes. During the consultation it is again stressed to Mr Bisic that he should have an HIV test and refrain from having penetrative sex, including oral, vaginal and anal, until his illness has cleared up. Dr Dolema also says that Mr Bisic's sexual partners ought to be informed and advised to consult their doctors. The doctor offers to assist in informing Mr Bisic's sexual partners but says Mr Bisic would have to tell him who they are. Mr Bisic responds, "Doc, you know one already, is Mr Shie who tell me to come to you. The only other one now is Sandra, and the last time when I tried to use a condom she started asking all sort of questions and say she used to get a rash whenever her first boyfriend used one." Dr Dolema remembers Mr Shie very well as one of his HIV-positive patients who has told him that he is celibate.

Discussion

The following discussions address the issues of professional conduct raised in the exercises. Other conclusions are possible.

◆ *Exercise 40*

Issues

- Does the nurse have a right to know about her husband's medical condition?
- Should the nurse have approached the laboratory without her husband's knowledge?
- Should the laboratory technician have given the information to the nurse?

Professional conduct

- Although the nurse is a concerned party and a health professional, she has no legal right to know her husband's medical information without his acquiescence and should not have approached the laboratory without his knowledge.
- A nurse is in a professional relationship with the laboratory that allows her to obtain information about patients. She has, however, misused this relationship in obtaining her husband's medical information without his permission and in a circumstance where he is not a patient.
- The laboratory technician, knowing the confidential and sensitive nature of the tests that are performed on donated blood, should not have treated this enquiry as a routine enquiry about a patient, particularly when the nurse identified herself as asking about her husband.
- The results of sensitive tests should not be given over the phone even to those whose voices are recognized.

◈ Exercise 41

Issues

- Can the proposed system ensure the confidentiality of patients' records?
- Does the notice of the hospital director answer the doctor's query?

Professional conduct

- Storage of confidential information on computers requires security measures to ensure that unauthorized people cannot access the data. The use of a national identity number to enable transactions between government departments appears to be a mechanism that can easily be accessed by unauthorized people, unless other security features are in place.
- It is entirely appropriate for the doctor to ask what safeguards are to be used to prevent unauthorized people from accessing medical records in a computer filing system and to determine the role of the national identity number in medical records.
- The hospital administrator seeks to explain the notice sent out from the medical records department but does not address the doctor's enquiry. The response, on the face of it, suggests that all government departments will have access to patient information.

◈ Exercise 42

Issues

- What is the mother's legal right to her son's medical information?
- Should the doctor accede to the boy's wishes or do as he suggested?

Professional conduct

- At 17, the boy has probably not reached the age of majority, and his parents are legally responsible for consenting to his treatment. On the other hand, the condition is a sexually transmitted disease, and it is probably lawful for a minor at this age to consent to sexual intercourse; thus he could be treated for a sexually acquired condition as a liberated minor.
- If the doctor decides to treat the boy as a liberated minor, the doctor must decide if it is in the minor's best interest that his parents do not know of the condition.
- The condition diagnosed requires more than the treatment of the acute illness; there is a need for better counselling than might be provided in the emergency room, including the issues of HIV testing and contact tracing, which may require consultation with specialist services. It may be difficult to accomplish all that is

necessary without some involvement of a concerned parent, and efforts must be made to have the boy agree to the involvement of a parent.

Exercise 43

Issues

- Should the doctor exclude the wife from the examination room?
- Does the wife have the right to know what is going on with her husband's illness?
- Should the doctor acquiesce with the patient's wish to deceive his wife?

Professional conduct

- The doctor may have perceived that the patient is not being allowed to speak for himself and has acted to give the patient the opportunity to do so.
- Exclusion from the examination room of a relative who is present with the patient's consent should be done only at the request of the patient or in the presence of someone like a nurse in attendance, who acts as an assistant and a chaperone.
- Although it is desirable that concerned relatives should know about a patient's illness, they have no right to know, and the patient's wishes should be adhered to unless the doctor is persuaded otherwise.

Exercise 44

Issues

- Should the employer have been given the patient's diagnosis?
- Should the doctor entertain the employer's request?
- Should the doctor accept the vouchers that were sent?

Professional conduct

- The employer should not have been privy to the diagnosis of the patient except with the express permission of the patient. The doctor has probably provided the diagnosis simply by copying an insurance claim form to the employer. Insurance claim forms are worded so that the patient agrees to have the diagnosis revealed in order to make a claim.
- It is professional misconduct to provide false certification. Presumably the doctor has already certified that the patient is fit to return to work, and to accede to the employer's request implies false or previously incorrect certification.
- There is normally nothing wrong in accepting promotional gifts, except when there is an expectation of professional misconduct in return. In the context of the

scenario, it could be construed that the vouchers are being sent to facilitate possible professional misconduct.

◆ Exercise 45

Issues

- Should the bank officer be privy to the reason for refusal of insurance coverage?
- Who has the responsibility, if any, to inform the patient about the results of tests done?
- What recourse, if any, has the patient?

Professional conduct

- The insurance company has received confidential information with the signed consent of the patient. Such information should not be divulged to any person or organization except with the patient's express consent.
- Regardless of any signed document for release of information, the examining doctor has a professional responsibility to inform the patient of any significant findings.
- Legal recourse for the client is difficult if, as expected, there is a signed release of her medical information to the insurance company. In the case of the examining doctor, a case of professional misconduct may or may not succeed, depending upon the arguments presented before the regulatory body.

Alternative conduct

- This situation is most likely to be encountered in the context of HIV testing, where insurance is refused for all persons testing positive. Clients should be given the opportunity to withdraw an application that cannot succeed.
- Doctors doing insurance examinations have other professional responsibilities. Thus, sensitive and crucial tests such as HIV positivity should be confirmed by repeat testing. The social and economic costs to the client are significant enough that doctors should ensure that such persons receive counselling.
- There should be legal sanctions for breaching confidentiality for anyone who handles sensitive medical information.

◆ Exercise 46

Issues

- Should the doctor answer queries from the press? If so, what should be said?
- Should the doctor take the cue from the daughter and proceed along similar lines?

Professional conduct

- The doctor should, where possible, discuss with the patient beforehand what information will be given to the press. If this has not been done, then the patient, or his or her surrogate, should be consulted and should give permission before the doctor talks to the press.
- The doctor should be wary of confirming or denying what relatives may have said to the press, since what is said may be inaccurate or incomplete. There may be directions that the relatives want the press to follow which have little to do with the actual situation.

Exercise 47

Issues

- Should patient information be revealed after death, even at the behest of a relative?
- Should a post-mortem be done in such a case, and how should the doctor respond to the press?

Professional conduct

- Patient information remains confidential after death and should be released only with the express consent of the next of kin.
- In the case of sudden, unexpected death, the coroner is responsible for determining the cause of death. The coroner may accept the opinion of an experienced and practised practitioner as to the cause of death and not perform a post-mortem. Therefore, the doctor should answer that the case has been reported to the coroner, as cases of sudden unexpected death require.

Exercise 48

Issues

- Is the government deceptive about its policy?
- Is the insurance company justified in screening for HIV and excluding applicants from coverage?
- Is Dr Too correct in asking the government for clarification?

Professional conduct

- If job applicants are being screened for HIV without being explicitly told that it is for health insurance purposes, and if the job must carry health insurance, then applicants are being deceived.

- Insurance companies have to examine risks, and therefore screening for various health risks is justified in providing coverage. However, when there is a group policy, the risks must be assessed on a group basis, and the insurance company should not seek to exclude individuals from the group.
- If Dr Too is doing screening on behalf of the government rather than the insurance company, clarification must be sought, for the role appears contrary to the stated government policy.
- Dr Too should clarify the position to the job applicants and have them sign a consent form for the screening.

◆ Exercise 49

Issues

- Is Dr Safer's policy of requiring HIV tests for all patients who are having major operations justifiable?
- Is the surgeon on duty justified in asking for an HIV test?
- Should the accident and emergency room officer have told Dr Safer about the request for the test?
- Can Dr Safer refuse to be treated by the surgeon on duty?

Professional conduct

- Policies should be based on evidence, and the testing requested should have a purpose – for example, does Dr Safer intend to exclude all HIV-positive patients from being operated on? The current evidence is that there has been no transmission of HIV in the operating theatre setting if personnel use normal universal precautions to avoid infection; the nearest incidents have been an accidental self-inflicted knife injury by a pathologist doing a post-mortem and the explosive splashing of a blood sample in the face of a laboratory worker. If Dr Safer is anticipating a possible major injury, then he and his assistants should be tested before operating on anyone.
- On the present evidence, there is no justification for the surgeon to ask for HIV testing on an emergency case, since there is a duty of care that must be exercised whatever the result of the test may be, and waiting for a result may compromise the care of the patient.
- If the officer thinks that a genuine request for HIV testing has been made, then it is his or her duty to inform the patient before the test is done and to obtain the patient's explicit consent.
- Dr Safer is within his rights as a patient to ask not to be treated by the surgeon on call; however, his pejorative remarks are unprofessional.

Exercise 50

Issues

- Should the doctor respond to the next of kin to preserve patient confidentiality?
- Can the doctor be truthful and still accede to the request of the patient's next of kin?

Professional conduct

- The doctor should ascertain the reason for the request. There are usually two reasons in such a situation: the avoidance of stigma and shame in the community and the ability to avoid an exclusion clause in an insurance matter. The family will require counselling to deal with the stigma, and it should be pointed out that there are possible legal consequences for a doctor who provides incorrect certification.
- The doctor could truthfully certify that death was due to liver failure as a result of a reaction to drugs. However, the use of the drug as a means of committing suicide is thereby obscured from those without a discerning eye. This reduces the ease and accuracy with which health information can be compiled and may represent an attempt to mislead the insurance company.
- If suicide is not certified and there is a request to provide additional information, the doctor should state whether, in his or her opinion, the drug was used to attempt suicide.

Exercise 51

Issues

- Does genital herpes or HIV infection fall into the category of fatal illnesses requiring third-party safeguards?
- Who are the third parties at risk for unknowingly acquiring HIV infection?
- Should Dr Dolema break the confidentiality of either of his patients?
- How should Dr Dolema deal with what he has been told about Sandra?

Professional conduct

- Dr Dolema has tried to preserve his patients' confidentiality while giving them advice to prevent the spread of HIV, herpes and any other sexually transmitted disease. He has also properly tried to persuade his patient to be tested for HIV but cannot force it upon the patient.
- Any sexually transmitted disease signals that the patient and his or her sexual partners are at risk of acquiring HIV infection. All three of the parties mentioned and other sexual partners of the three are at risk and must be so considered.

- Dr Dolema has good grounds to breach Mr Shie's confidentiality after confronting him with the fact that Mr Shie is indeed having sexual relations with Mr Bisic while stating that he is celibate.
- Sandra may have an allergic reaction to latex condoms or may be giving an excuse for not using them. She also may be interpreting the man's suggestion of using a condom as an indicator of his possible illness, including HIV status, and is testing out his responses. A way must be found to have Sandra counselled and examined. If Mr Bisic proves to be HIV-positive and fails to inform Sandra, she should be warned by the doctor.

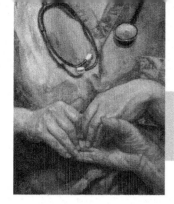

CHAPTER '7'

Consent to Treatment

C   *onsent* is an agreement to permit someone to do something. It can be implied, given verbally or given in writing. *Treatment* is anything done in the course of addressing an illness. Those entitled to treat patients are defined in the laws governing the health professions; however, such laws do not prevent the application of home remedies by people who do not claim to be health professionals.

Any patient who is legally and mentally competent has an absolute right to consent to, or refuse, anything that is done to him or her in the context of health care. This includes treatments that appear to be minor and not a threat to one's well-being, those that may appear trivial to health-care staff, and those that put the patient's life at risk.

Competence

Legal competence resides in any adult who is capable of understanding the matter to which he or she is asked to consent. Adulthood is defined in any given jurisdiction by the attainment of the age of majority as defined by law. In most jurisdictions this is 18 years, and in some it is 21 years. In the United Kingdom the age is 16 years for matters pertaining to medical treatment but is otherwise 18 years. If an adult patient is unable to consent – if, for example, the patient is in a coma – the next of kin or the person in charge of an institution responsible for the person may legally consent on the patient's behalf [see Exercise 52].

Mental competence is assumed to exist unless the person has an illness which significantly impairs mental capacity. A person's mental capacity is clearly impaired if he or she is in a coma; a person may be conscious but incoherent or disoriented for a variety of causes; or there may be a severe enough mental illness to cause a person to be judged by mental health professionals to be incapable of making a coherent judgement.

Mental illness is usually dealt with under specific laws and regulations, which define the way a person's competence is determined and how a mentally incompetent person's legal affairs will be handled. For example, in Barbados, under the Mental Health Act, a person who is involuntarily admitted to the psychiatric hospital can be deemed by the senior psychiatrist in charge of the institution to be incapable of giving consent.

Whenever mental incompetence is established, consent has to be given on behalf of the patient by the next of kin or by the legal guardian, who is either a person appointed by the court or an institution within the definition of the law. Anything done to a patient who cannot personally give consent must be clearly demonstrable to be in the patient's best interest rather than that of the guardian or the institution [see Exercise 53].

Age of consent

Minors, who are persons below the age of majority [see *Legal competence* above], require consent to be given for them by one of their parents or their legal guardian. However, minors have the capacity to consent to treatment in certain instances that are established by precedent in case law or by statute. Thus, although the legal age of consent for sexual intercourse (16 years old in most instances) is lower than the age of majority, a person that age normally does not have the legal capacity to consent to the treatment of a sexually transmitted disease or its consequences, if such consent becomes an issue. However, as the result of statute law, a 16-year-old in Barbados can consent, independently of her parents, to a termination of pregnancy under the Medical Termination of Pregnancy Act (1983); there is a similar provision in the laws of Guyana. However, it is not clear that the same young woman would be able to consent to a caesarean section being performed if that became necessary. After the birth of her child, the 16-year-old mother can give consent for the treatment of her child but is not entitled in law to give consent for her own treatment unless she is treated as a liberated minor. In the United Kingdom, the Family Law Reform Act (1969) established that minors 16 and 17 years of age can consent to any medical therapy without the consent of their parents.

The *liberated minor* was established as a legal concept in 1985 by a court decision in the United Kingdom known as the Gillick case [*Gillick v. West Norfolk Area Health Authority*, 3 A.E.R. 402 (1985)]. It provides that the wishes of a minor can override the wishes of the parents under certain circumstances. The specific case was about the provision of contraception to a minor, but it established certain general ground rules about minors being able to consent for themselves:

1) The minor must understand the advice being given.
2) The minor does not wish the parent to know about the illness or treatment and cannot be persuaded otherwise.

3) The minor is likely to continue with the risk behaviour or illness, and it is likely to produce harm to the minor.
4) The best interest of the minor would be served, in spite of parental disapproval.

Whenever there is doubt about the legal course to be followed, health professionals should seek legal advice or obtain a court order [see Exercise 54].

Informed consent

Although the term *informed consent* is commonly associated with research, all consent should be informed. The term refers to the requirement that patients should know and understand what they have consented to. This means that the diagnosis, general nature of the procedure proposed, anticipated benefits and risks, and any alternatives should be explained. Explanations should be in terms that the patient can understand, rather than terms that are clear only to other health professionals. In explaining informed consent, a judge has exhorted surgeons to "Advise patients of those material facts, risks, complications and alternatives to surgery that a reasonable person in the patient's situation would consider significant in deciding whether to have an operation" [*Rowinsky v. Sperling*, 681 A.2n 785 (Pa. 1996)].

Forms of consent include those that are implied, oral or written.

• If a person offers to have a blood sample taken, consent to do the test is implied. However, if the person discovers that a test was performed which was not something that he or she wanted done, then the "implied consent" is invalidated.
• Oral consent should be obtained for tests or "minor" procedures depending on the seriousness of the expected result or risk. Harm to a patient can be psychosocial – for example, diagnosing a condition, such as HIV infection, that carries a significant stigma in the community, or diagnosing a malignancy, which causes fear in the patient. In such instances there is no place for implied consent, although oral consent may suffice.
• In surgical procedures the risk of physical harm is obvious; therefore, written consent is insisted upon. However, it must be remembered that such documents are only indicative of the patient's awareness of the event and cannot be seen as legal sanction to do something that may harm the patient. Informed consent with a written record is necessary in clinical situations where events, no matter how rarely they occur, may have a serious and permanent effect on the patient. There is a fine line between outlining all the risks of a procedure and calling to the patient's attention the possibility of unusual but specific events that may occur. For example, it is prudent to warn every patient undergoing parotid surgery about the possibility of facial nerve palsy, whereas it is not necessary to stress, unless asked, that the patient may suffer a cardiac arrest during the procedure or the recovery period.

Refusal to consent

Any competent patient, parent of a minor, or legal guardian can refuse any investigation or treatment offered. Such refusal can be overridden only by a court of law. A patient can refuse treatment at anytime, even after a procedure has been started. It is wise to have refusal of advice recorded and witnessed [see Exercise 55].

Treatment without consent

Any doctor may act in the best interest of a patient in an emergency life-threatening situation. Nonetheless, anything done to a competent patient without the patient's consent, whether it is an emergency or not, is an assault in law. The remedies available to the patient who has been treated without consent include a criminal charge of battery and civil action for negligence.

Consent for research

The term *informed consent* has come to be associated with interventional research on human subjects, and implies a written record of the explanation given about the intervention to be employed, its benefits and its risks [see Exercise 56].

Situations of uncertainty

Situations of uncertainty may exist when legal parameters are not well defined, because laws vary in different countries or because practice varies between institutions. In such situations the practitioner should seek advice from the available legal or ethical resources. In hospital practice, two well-recognized situations of uncertainty involve organ donation and withdrawal of life support.

Organ donation

A competent person can consent to donate an organ to another person. In some countries it is unlawful to traffic in human organs, whereas in others the practice occurs. Organ donation after death should be done within a legal framework, where one exists. In countries with no specific law governing cadaveric organ donation, consent should be obtained from the coroner and the next of kin. However, it could be considered unethical to procure organs for donation if the patient, when competent, had clearly expressed a wish otherwise [see Exercise 57].

Brain death

Similar legal and ethical considerations to those above apply to the question of cessation of artificial life support for people who are determined to be "brain-dead". Some countries have a statute that defines brain death; most do not. However, the concept of brain death can be established in common law by standards acceptable to the broad body of medical practitioners. It is therefore prudent, where a brain-death statute does not exist, and in many instances where it does, to obtain the agreement of the next of kin with any decision to cease life support in a patient diagnosed as brain-dead [see Exercise 58].

Futility of treatment

In some situations where treatment has been judged to be futile, consideration is given to withdrawal of life-supporting treatment. Consent to do so lies with the patient or legal guardian. Patients are not usually in a condition to make the decision at the time it arises, but many people have sought to retain control by previously signing a "living will". Doctors and guardians often evade the decision for withdrawal of life support by consenting to a do-not-resuscitate (DNR) order. Living wills and DNR orders should be considered as indicative of a patient's wishes but should not override clinical judgement. Good clinical judgement should not encourage exercises in futility [see Exercise 59].

Exercises 52 to 59

The following scenarios are based on events in practice. Identify the ethical and legal issues and state whether the conduct of the professionals was correct and why. If the professional conduct was not correct, state what it should have been. Discussion follows the exercises.

◈ Exercise 52

An 80-year-old woman attends the outpatient department complaining of abdominal pain, the cause of which is diagnosed as a large abdominal aortic aneurysm. The surgeon advises that she should have an operation since the pain indicates that it could rupture. The patient asks, "Doc, you think I will be able to stand the operation?" The surgeon responds that although the operation is a risky one, it is the only way to get rid of the pain, but that if the aneurysm ruptures she will almost certainly die. Her daughter, who accompanied her, interrupts and says, "She is too old for an operation – I will not allow it!"

◈ Exercise 53

A 79-year-old man is accompanied by his neighbour to the operating theatre, where he is booked to have a hernia operation under local anaesthesia. The nurse is filling out the anaesthesia and consent forms and notices that the neighbour interrupts to answer most of the questions. When it comes to signing the consent form, the nurse calls the surgeon and says, "I am not sure that Mr Feebel should sign the consent form. He does not seem to be all there."

◈ Exercise 54

A 16-year-old girl is seen with a fracture of her forearm and is advised that it requires reduction under general anaesthesia. The nurse tells her she must get a parent to sign the consent form. The girl replies, "I don't live with my mother, and my father lives overseas." On being told she should obtain her mother's consent anyway, she says, "We don't speak, and anyway I signed my own consent when I had the operation last time."

◈ Exercise 55

A 60-year-old woman has come as an outpatient to have an operation done under local anaesthesia. She signs the consent form and is taken to the operating theatre. When she is told that she is about to be injected with the local anaesthetic, she protests that she does not want any injection. She is told that this is how the local anaesthetic is given, and she responds that she was told she wouldn't be going to sleep and that the area would be deadened so she wouldn't feel the operation, but nothing was said about an injection. She remains unpersuaded and declares that she does not want the operation anymore.

Exercise 56

Dr Extent has obtained approval to carry out a clinical trial comparing a new diabetes medication with one that is currently in use. He has given his assistant the protocol to read and has briefed the assistant on the procedures to be carried out during the trial. The assistant asks for copies of the consent form, and Dr Extent responds, "Don't bother with that, the patients need treatment anyway and they might not agree if they know it is an experiment they are in."

Exercise 57

A 58-year-old businessman with chronic renal failure is advised by his doctor to see if any of his relatives will donate one of their kidneys to him. He responds that he has already discussed it and they all claim to have some problem, and the relatives have pointed out that one of his friends paid to get a kidney donated. He asks his doctor if that could be arranged. The doctor responds that buying a kidney is not allowed in this country but he knows of a colleague in another country that will arrange it, if the businessman is prepared to go there for the operation.

Exercise 58

Newspaper article:

> *Doctor Removes Ventilator from a Patient, Gives It to Relative of a Colleague*
> A nurse who wishes to remain anonymous reported to this newspaper that a 75-year-old man who had a stroke and was on a ventilator for the past week was suddenly removed from the ventilator and died shortly thereafter. Within the hour the 80-year-old uncle of a doctor was admitted to the intensive care unit and put on the ventilator. When contacted, the doctor in charge of the unit said that the ventilator was removed from the patient because he was brain-dead. The children of the patient claim that they were not told anything about their father being brain-dead or the ventilator being removed.

Exercise 59

A 45-year-old man with a family history of sudden death complains of a severe headache, collapses and is admitted to the hospital with a diagnosis of a ruptured berry aneurysm. He is seen by the neurosurgeon, who, after investigation, advises that the aneurysm be clipped. His wife signs the consent form and the surgery is done. After a week the man remains unresponsive on the ventilator. His wife, after asking about the chances of recovery, asks the surgeon to remove her husband from the ventilator "as it was always his wish not to have to live like that".

Discussion

The following discussions address the issues of professional conduct raised in the exercises. Other conclusions are possible.

◆ Exercise 52

Issues

- Has the doctor revealed all of the information necessary for the patient to make an informed decision?
- Does the daughter have the right to veto an operation being performed on her mother?
- Is the patient competent to make the decision about the operation?

Professional conduct

- The doctor should give all pertinent information and explain the risks of the procedure to allow the patient or guardian to make an informed decision. In this case, it appears that the doctor has given the information necessary, although not in sufficient detail for the patient to judge the risk of not having the operation.
- The doctor has answered truthfully when asked additional questions by the patient. There is a fine judgement to be made about explaining all of the risks of a procedure, which might deter a patient from following advice.
- The daughter makes a common misjudgement that "old" patients should not be operated on except when absolutely necessary. The doctor therefore must explain in detail the risks of not doing the procedure, if the relative is to make a decision as a surrogate.
- In this case, there is nothing to suggest that the patient is mentally impaired, and the daughter has no legal competence to make the decision not to operate. However, the patient may feel more comfortable going along with her daughter's opinion, particularly if she is dependent on her children financially or otherwise for care and support.
- The doctor must determine whether the patient is mentally competent to make the decision for herself and, if so, point out to the patient and the relatives that the decision is the patient's to make.

◆ Exercise 53

Issues

- Is the nurse competent to make the determination of mental competence?
- Given that the procedure is to be carried out under local anaesthesia, is the risk enough to insist that legal competence to consent be established?
- Should the neighbour be asked to sign the consent form?
- Has consent been established once the patient has voluntarily come for the operation?

Professional conduct

- The nurse is in a position to make a judgement as to the competence of the patient but cannot determine it with certainty; she therefore defers the judgement to the doctor in charge of the patient. The doctor in charge may take the decision about the mental competence of the patient, but if in doubt the doctor should seek a specialist referral. If the patient had a next of kin or a legal guardian available, then that person could be asked to sign the consent form. In the case described, the neighbour is probably not the legal guardian and therefore should not be asked to sign, no matter how close the relationship with the patient may appear.
- Legal competence to consent should always be established in non-emergency situations, even when the risks are small. In an emergency situation, the doctor in charge can undertake the responsibility to treat without consent.
- Although consent is implied if a patient voluntarily attends for a procedure to be done, this does not obviate the need to obtain written approval for invasive procedures.

◆ Exercise 54

Issues

- What is the age of majority in the jurisdiction?
- Is there any circumstance that allows a minor to sign his or her own consent form?
- In the absence of parents, does the minor have a legal guardian?

Professional conduct

- In most jurisdictions the age of majority, at which one can sign one's own consent form, is 18 years or older. The nurse is therefore probably correct in asking the girl to have her mother sign.
- There are exceptions established by statute or case law in which minors can consent to operation, and these will apply in the particular jurisdiction.

- In the absence of parents a minor should have a legal guardian, who may be a relative, a court-appointed guardian, or a spouse in those jurisdictions where minors can be married. In the absence of all of these, the institution or the doctor can accept the responsibility, particularly in emergency situations.

◆ Exercise 55

Issues

- Can consent be withdrawn after the consent form is signed?
- Has the woman been misled about the nature of the procedure?

Professional conduct

- Consent can be withdrawn at any time, even after a procedure has begun. The health-care professionals should try to persuade the patient to carry on, but failing that, they must stop the procedure as safely as possible while keeping the patient fully informed.
- Procedures that are considered routine by a health professional may loom large for the patient. The patient has clearly not received certain information that was crucial to her. This problem can be averted if health-care staff spend more time with patients so that their questions can be answered, and by providing written and illustrative material for patients to review before any procedure occurs.

◆ Exercise 56

Issues

- Is there any justification for concealing a new treatment from a patient?
- How should an assistant respond to a breach in a research protocol?

Professional conduct

- There can be no justification for not obtaining some form of consent to interventional research. If there is any justification for withholding information from the subject of research, it must be argued before and approved by the body approving the research protocol. If a change in practice is considered desirable after the protocol has been approved, then the proposed change should be submitted for approval.
- Anyone involved in research should follow the approved protocol and point out any breaches to supervisors. If a participant in research cannot resolve an issue with supervisors, they should seek legal or ethical advice, as appropriate.

Exercise 57

Issues

- What is wrong with buying organs for transplantation?
- If it is illegal or unethical to buy organs in the area where the doctor practises, should it be recommended as acceptable elsewhere?

Professional conduct

- The ethical arguments against buying organs are that the practice exploits the poor and that when it comes to vital organs, there is the possibility that health professionals may make faulty judgements regarding whether the patient is brain-dead and the organs are therefore available. Although donating blood does not threaten the donor's survival as does donation of other organs, the practice of buying blood from donors has led to a variety of abuses.
- Unacceptable practices may be determined by law or by an ethical code of conduct within the profession. Doctors should not recommend that a patient go to another jurisdiction for treatment unless they satisfy themselves that the recommended measure is lawful and ethical in the country being recommended.

Exercise 58

Issues

- Should a health professional make reports to the press about problems in the institution in which he or she works?
- Does the doctor have the right to remove a ventilator from a patient without the consent of the relatives?
- Should doctors make decisions about the allocation of scarce resources for one patient or another?

Professional conduct

- Professionals should not see the press as the first point of call to address concerns. However, the institution must have credible mechanisms that staff can use to address ethical or legal problems without the fear of being victimized.
- Life-support measures, and in particular ventilation, carry an important technical as well as emotional place in the minds of professionals and laypersons. Therefore, the cessation of ventilation must be a carefully considered decision which is shared with and justified to all those involved – patients, relatives and caregivers.

- In jurisdictions where brain death is accepted within the law, the doctor's right to stop all treatment is supportable in law. However, death is seen by most persons as the cessation of the heartbeat, and it is therefore prudent to explain to all involved how the decision about death was arrived at, and why life-support measures are being withdrawn.
- Doctors and others involved in health care are often faced with decisions that involve the allocation of scarce resources, and should be prepared to explain their decisions if challenged. When the situations involve immediate issues of life or death, then justification as well as an explanation may be required.

◆ Exercise 59

Issues

- Should the wife's request for withdrawal of life support be honoured?
- Should the reported statement of the patient have any bearing on the doctor's decision?
- Are there any determinations that can help the doctor reach a decision?

Professional conduct

- The wife, as the person legally responsible for the incapacitated patient, has acted in that capacity in giving consent for the operation and now has the legal authority to request the cessation of treatment. The request should be honoured unless the physician in charge of the patient feels that continued therapy will lead to recovery. If such a disagreement exists and the patient's surrogate cannot be persuaded otherwise, the parties have recourse to the courts.
- When there is disagreement among the parties about whether life support should be stopped, the patient's prior wishes will be very influential in any decision, in court or otherwise. The patient's history, statements from close friends and relatives and the presence of any documentation such as a living will will also have an influence on the decision.
- Physicians faced with uncertain outcomes should seek second opinions and any investigations or consultations that could help in making a determination. For example, in a case like this it would be crucial to determine whether the patient is brain-dead, and, if so, the physician should adhere to the surrogate's wishes.

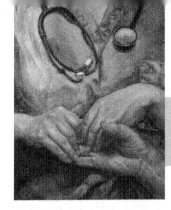

Life and Death

Health-care professionals are trained to preserve life and to help their patients maintain a state of physical and emotional well-being. The beginning and the end of life offer challenges to the basic tenets of health care when professionals have to make decisions about the preservation of life, particularly when it appears that an acceptable state of physical and emotional well-being cannot be maintained.

Despite our technological sophistication, the beginning and the end of life continue to have a mystical quality that is intimately bound to religious beliefs. However, given the diversity of religious doctrines, it is natural that ethical viewpoints on these defining points of life will differ; as a consequence, there is little uniformity between jurisdictions in the laws related to the beginning and the end of life. It is therefore incumbent on health professionals to be conversant with the issues involved and the laws governing the practice of the profession in their jurisdiction.

In many areas, technological advances are occurring too fast for society to keep up ethically: it takes time and consideration to reach the ethical consensus and legal constructs required to deal with the possibilities created by biomedical technology.

The most important ethical and legal issues related to the beginning of life are termination of pregnancy, *in vitro* fertilization, surrogate motherhood, stem cell research and cloning. Ethical issues that arise at the end of life include the definition of death, the right to die, the use of the body after death and the preservation of civil and legal rights after death.

The beginning of life

Different religious doctrines answer the question "When does life begin?" in different ways. As a consequence, legal definitions vary depending on the predominant religious influence that is brought to bear on legislators. In the past generation, the influence of women who believe they should have the right to determine the fate of their own bodies and the pregnancy they may bear has had an important impact on legislation.

Termination of pregnancy

Viewpoints vary widely on the termination of pregnancy. At one end of the spectrum are those who view life as beginning at conception; it is the view of the Roman Catholic Church that there should be no impediment placed in the way of conception and that there is no justification for ending a pregnancy. At the other end of the spectrum are those who believe that the life of a foetus is not significant until the foetus can exist independent of the womb. There are, of course, other perspectives in between. It is unlikely that there will be universal resolution of these viewpoints, for people's ethical and moral positions are most influenced by their faith, even when the law takes a different position. This can be a dilemma for health-care professionals, who have a duty to obey the law in the jurisdiction in which they practise even when their religious beliefs are contrary to that law. In some countries the termination of a pregnancy is against the law under any circumstance, whereas in others the procedure may be carried out under defined circumstances, which may include social factors, the mother's health and the stage of the pregnancy [see Exercise 60].

In vitro fertilization

In vitro fertilization consists of the fertilization of an ovum in the laboratory and the implantation of the developing embryo into the womb. Apart from the risks of the procedure, which must be explained, this reproductive technology incorporates various sensitive issues with ethical implications. These issues include the choice of donor of the sperm or ovum, confidentiality of the donor, whether the "parents" are the biological or the legal parents, the use of surrogate mothers, the fate of unused embryos, and cloning.

Persons who are unable to contribute their own genetic material to the process of having a child may have relatives or friends who voluntarily donate sperm or ova, or may choose a donor of sperm or ova from a list of anonymous donors who are paid for the service. Donors are described to the clients in physical and occupational terms, and, particularly in small communities, the question may arise of whether the donor's identity can be determined. In addition, the possibility exists that multiple clients may choose the same donor and create multiple genetic siblings. As genetic studies become more common for the identification of paternity and for diagnosing some diseases, the potential for loss of donor anonymity increases, particularly when children become curious about their genetic parent. To reduce the possibility of conflict, great care should be taken to keep the donors and recipients of genetic material anonymous in relation to each other [see Exercise 61].

Maintaining the confidentiality and anonymity of the donor is more difficult when the donor is a woman, because medical and surgical procedures are involved and because a contract for payment may be made between the client and the donor. Donation of sperm by a man, in contrast, does not require a personal contract [see Exercise 62].

Children will naturally be curious about their biological parents, and there is a possibility of conflict should the genetic donors be identified. Since fertilized ova are allowed to develop before implantation to ensure that normal cellular division is occurring, the potential exists for the implantation of the wrong embryo. Procedures to guard against this possibility must be zealously developed and followed [see Exercise 63].

Surrogate motherhood

Whenever a surrogate mother carries a pregnancy to completion and then gives up the infant under a previous contractual obligation, the possibility of major conflict exists. The surrogate may or may not have contributed some of the genetic material and may have psychologically bonded with the infant during the pregnancy. The process of giving up the infant is not akin to a promise to give up an infant for adoption, for that promise can be simply withdrawn. In these arrangements, the surrogate may have been paid for the service of going through the pregnancy, and the genetic material may not be her own. Contracts for surrogacy have come under dispute in court when the surrogate changes her mind about giving up the infant, and laws vary on this matter. Where specific law does not exist, the birth mother is considered the legal mother. Specific laws related to surrogacy exist in some jurisdictions, including a law in France that excludes post-menopausal women from being involved in the process – a restriction that is not present in other jurisdictions. In the State of New York it is against the law to be involved in any compensation arrangements for surrogacy [see Exercise 64].

The use of embryos

The freezing of embryos for future use is a frequent outcome of the process of *in vitro* fertilization, because often more ova are fertilized than are initially implanted. Such embryos, when no longer needed, are destroyed or used for research purposes. The fate and ownership of these embryos have become matters of legal dispute; in one instance, after the genetic parents died in an accident, a claim was made that the embryos were the inheritors of the parents' estate and should be implanted into a surrogate to make the claim a reality.

Research on embryos has become a matter of great debate, for there are strongly held and apparently irreconcilable ethical viewpoints on the nature of the embryo. Some people maintain that an embryo is a human being and should not be subjected to experimentation, whereas others argue that an embryo has not reached a sufficient stage of development to be defined as a human being. Those who argue in favour of doing stem cell research point out that the embryos would be destroyed in any case, and that they have the potential for enabling the development of medical treatment for a variety of conditions.

Cloning

Cloning is a process whereby the genetic material in the nucleus of an ovum is replaced by the nuclear material of another person and activated without fertilization. If the activated ovum develops normally, it produces a carbon copy of the person whose nuclear material was used. Cloning has been achieved in animals, and so far cloned animals have had many developmental defects and experienced premature aging. Many fear that cloning may be employed to attempt to produce a "master race". Historically, such concepts have been articulated before, by regimes that have eventually proven to be aggressive and incompatible with the human-rights values developed in modern times.

Some people claim that cloning is natural, in that identical twins are the result of nature's act of cloning. The flaw in this argument is that identical twins are not the product of a previously existing person, they do not represent an *intention* to interfere with genetic diversity, and they exist contemporaneously. There is no model in nature for the sequential existence of persons with the same genetic make-up.

Arguments have been raised for using cloning to produce human tissue for treatment purposes. How this would be achieved, in terms of organ production, is not yet clear and remains a subject of debate and ongoing research. The cloning of stem cells for the purpose of treatment of the individual would seem to have few ethical drawbacks, but it is objectionable to some religions that have a fundamental objection to any use of embryonic tissue [see Exercise 65].

Choosing who will live

Choosing who will live is a responsibility that sometimes has to be faced by health professionals, and it often places the professional's technological judgement in conflict with the choice of a parent or patient – a choice usually made primarily with religious guidance.

Infant versus mother

Having to choose between the life of an infant and that of its mother is increasingly rare. If faced with the choice between saving her own life and saving that of her unborn infant, a pregnant woman is entitled to make the decision, and usually seeks guidance and support from her religion and her family. Her choice may be challenged by health professionals or the state, depending on the decision and the prevailing mores of the time. Such challenges, if unresolved, may have to be decided in the court.

A mother's choice of her life over that of her infant may be challenged by a state that does not allow abortion under any circumstance, as in those countries whose laws reflect the doctrines of the Roman Catholic Church. In most jurisdictions, the law allows for the termination of a pregnancy in order to save the life of the mother, and any challenge under the law would be to the technical judgement of the health professionals as to whether the mother's life is in fact endangered. The challenge may come from the acknowledged father or from community groups opposed to abortion. Such challenges can only be determined in a court of law.

A mother's choice of the life of her infant over her own appears to be an artefact of the increasing sophistication of anaesthetic and life-support techniques. Nevertheless, such a judgement on the mother's part would be open to challenge by her family, the health-care establishment and the state, all of whom may feel that her life is crucial to the well-being of other children and that she may have the opportunity to bear another child. This choice has usually had to be made under emergency circumstances, and it is difficult to have the matter resolved by the court. The choice therefore remains with the professional, who should take a course of action that gives both the mother and her infant a chance at life, the balance of probabilities being left to the technology available at the time [see Exercise 66].

Too many foetuses

Advances in the treatment of infertility have led to the possibility that a large number of fertilized ova may implant and develop. Foetuses will compete for resources, and consideration may be given to the abortion of some foetuses in order for others to survive. The possibility that such a decision will have to be made should be addressed in the counselling process and in the prior agreements made when undertaking such procedures.

The abnormal foetus

An infant born with congenital abnormalities may experience a diminished quality of life and tax the family's emotional and economic resources. Abortion of an abnormal foetus has thus become an option in some jurisdictions. A pregnant woman who becomes infected with rubella is likely to bear a deaf child with congenital cardiac disease, and in jurisdictions where abortions are allowed, a woman in that situation may be offered an abortion on the grounds that the infant may be affected.

The ethics of aborting an abnormal or possibly abnormal foetus have been challenged not only on the grounds of opposition to abortion but also on the grounds that the child's abnormalities should be treated or the facilities provided to cope with the child's disabilities. Advances in the prevention and treatment of congenital abnormalities, including intrauterine surgery, have diminished the justification for abortion on the grounds of abnormalities. It is therefore incumbent on professionals who set about to diagnose abnormalities in a foetus to counsel the parents before they do so and to have a plan of action in the event an abnormality is diagnosed [see Exercise 67].

Choosing a gender

Technological advances in ultrasound diagnosis have enabled the identification of the gender of a foetus at an early stage. In some cultures this has led to abortion of foetuses (usually females), even though the law of the country may forbid it. Before identifying and revealing the gender of a foetus, the prudent health professional should discuss the matter with the parents to ensure that gender is not an issue for them. Gender is not an abnormality, and there can be no ethical or legal justification to terminate a pregnancy on that ground alone.

Siamese twins

In modern medical practice, Siamese twins who are born are investigated to consider the possibility of their separation. There are instances where the technical judgement is made that separation is possible only at the expense of the life of one of the twins. Where the health professionals and the parents cannot agree, usually on religious grounds, the impasse can only be settled by the court.

In the case of young children, judges can usually be relied upon to accept the word of the professionals who state that inaction would lead to death while action could lead to life. In a case before the court in the United Kingdom, doctors asked the court to allow them to separate Siamese twins against the wishes of the parents, knowing that the procedure would result in the certain death of one child but would save the life of the other. The parents had stated that they could not agree to the taking of the life of one of their children and that God's will should prevail for both. The court found for the doctors, accepting the argument that one twin would die from its abnormalities and cause the death of the other.

The end of life: death and dying

Decisions about care at the end of life are a measure of the availability of resources, and consequently such decisions are bound up in local circumstances. Choices have to be made regarding who will receive long-term haemodialysis, scarce donor organs for transplantation and expensive drugs for the treatment of diseases such as cancer and AIDS. When resources are available to either individuals or groups, there are usually no ethical or legal issues except in the case of organ procurement.

Organ procurement

In all countries, the donation of human organs is a voluntary exercise, and in most countries it is considered unethical to use monetary or other incentives to procure the donation of organs. In some countries, including the United Kingdom, doctors have been struck off the register to practise for being involved in the trafficking of human organs, while in others – for example, India – no legal sanction has been imposed for such trafficking [see Exercise 57].

The ethical argument against trafficking in human organs is that it invariably targets the poor and uneducated, who may not have a clear understanding of the risks they face, and who are unlikely to have any recourse should the risks materialize. The rationale for allowing trafficking is that both parties derive benefit; that the donor has made an informed choice; that it expands the pool of available donor organs, thereby benefiting more persons in need; and that in many circumstances blood for transfusion is bought and sold. The logical outcome of a legal traffic in human organs is the development of a market where the highest bidder wins, leading to other situations involving the trafficking of human beings, whether alive or dead.

Since donor organs are scarce in relation to the need, decisions about who will receive organs have to be made on grounds that are acceptable to the community. The criteria most often used are the chance of success, based on immunological matching; the assessed urgency of the need; and the chance of recovery, based on the patient's condition and age and available outcome data. These criteria are best applied through the development of institutional protocols rather than through relying on the judgement of the individual physicians who are directly involved in the treatment of the patients.

Terminal illness

Terminal illness describes a pathological state that cannot be controlled or altered to the extent that the death of a person can be stopped. It is therefore essential that an accurate diagnosis be made and the natural history of the condition be assessed to reach the conclusion that the patient is reaching the end of life.

Medical, nursing and other health-care professionals are trained to keep patients alive, and in this they are aided by advances in biomedical technology. Many professionals find it difficult to accept the death of a patient without first applying all available resources to try to prevent it. Some health-care professionals may make the "diagnosis" of dying reluctantly and may enter into conflict with others, including the patient, over the course of treatment that should be taken.

Dying is a process of physical or mental deterioration leading to death within minutes, hours or days rather than weeks or months. It is an assessment made by knowledgeable and experienced health-care professionals, but there are no clear diagnostic parameters, and it is open to wide interpretation by patients, relatives and others. Without a clear definition, there is potential for conflict on what should be done at this stage of the patient's life.

When caregivers and patients (and relatives) differ in their assessment of whether a patient is terminally ill, or how the terminal illness should be dealt with, a number of issues and proposals have to be considered. Some of the issues are the use and cessation of life-support measures, a living will, euthanasia, and the benefits and harm of narcotic analgesia.

Persistent vegetative state

A persistent vegetative state is one in which there is sufficient cortical brain damage to preclude any expectation that the patient will regain consciousness. However, there may be sufficient neurological activity to enable spontaneous movement that may support unaided respiration. There are no confirmatory tests for this state, and the diagnosis is made by excluding recoverable causes of a coma and ensuring by observation over a period of time that neurological recovery will not occur.

Death

Death is the endpoint of the process of dying and is diagnosed and certified by a medical practitioner. However, death is not always preceded by dying, for there are sudden and unexpected deaths. In addition, there is the concept of brain death, in which the commonly accepted indicators of cessation of heartbeat and breathing have not occurred and the patient may be said to be "dying" although dead by professional assessment and/or legal definition.

Brain death is diagnosed when there is evidence of an irreversible lack of brain activity but the heart continues to beat. It is an anomalous state, in that the patient is dying while already dead. From a legal viewpoint, brain death cannot be certified by the issue of a death certificate but can inform a decision about withdrawal of life support from the patient or use of the "dead" patient's organs for transplantation.

Patients who are brain-dead can look remarkably normal except that they are being ventilated. Both staff and relatives must be made aware of the patient's condition and of how the diagnosis was made by the doctors in charge. If the patient's actual state is not made clear, staff or relatives may feel that some wrong is being perpetrated if life support is withdrawn.

Life-support measures

Death is about to occur when the heart has ceased to beat and the patient ceases to breathe, or when either of these circumstances is imminent. Resuscitation can be done to reverse or prevent death. In some instances, hypoxic brain damage may leave the patient without conscious existence and dependent on life-support measures. In some cases, the doctors' judgement is that there is no prospect of the patient's ever being anything more than a "vegetable". Being a "vegetable" is feared by both patients and their relatives and is seen by most health-care professionals as a failure of the resuscitative process. Professionals may also consider treatment of such a state to be a misuse of resources, both human and physical. The decision to resuscitate can therefore depend on a number of factors, which cannot be reasonably balanced in most emergency situations. As a result, many institutions have developed protocols to guide staff in the use of resuscitative measures. Such protocols must take into account

- the diagnosis and prognosis of the patient,
- the availability of human and physical resources,
- the expressed wishes of the patient or legal guardian, and
- the legal and ethical framework of the country and the institution.

The diagnosis and prognosis of the patient are determined by the physicians to whose care the patient is entrusted. Other health professionals will have views on the patient's condition and may not agree with the doctor in charge or have time, in an emergency situation, to fully explore that doctor's views. Prudently, protocols usually establish broad rather than exact parameters for the institution of resuscitation measures. The practice of making DNR orders may not work well, since most health-care staff are unwilling to undertake the responsibility of inaction on the basis of someone else's opinion, particularly when such orders have no legal force. The living will represents an attempt to add greater legal force to such orders and to prevent the initiation of unwanted treatment measures.

When to cease life-support treatment is a difficult decision, for medicine is still an imperfect science, and one does not know when the judgement that a patient is dying will prove to be faulty. In making such decisions, therefore, the patient's or legal guardian's wishes have to be taken into account. A legal guardian may be a parent, spouse or other next of kin, or, for those patients who are judged to be incapable of making a decision and where no next of kin is available, a guardian appointed by a court or the head of the treating institution. Although the doctor in charge has the final responsibility for deciding whether to continue or withdraw life-support measures, it is wise to take into account the views of others on the health-care team and to seek other opinions. As much as possible, second opinions should be sought from people who have not had anything to do with the care of the patient, for it is very difficult not to be biased by one's previous decisions. In many places, "second" opinions are in the form of opinions from or consultations with ethicists and ethical committees.

Because so many people need to be consulted, the difficult decision to cease treatment may take time to reach, and the same ground may have to be gone over repeatedly. Even when the decision is made, it is often not the end of the matter, for there are other decisions that become problematic – for example, what constitutes treatment. The most obvious treatment modalities are ventilatory support, medication (which includes cardiac support drugs, antibiotics and analgesics), intravenous nutrition and maintenance of fluid balance.

All of these treatment modalities have been tested in court when doctors have failed to resolve the differences between their point of view and that of relatives, the patient and, in some instances, other members of the health-care team. It is not possible to rely solely on the idea that the health-care team knows best, for there are many uncertainties in knowledge, and confounding events may occur in the course of a patient's care [see Exercise 68].

Ventilators

Ventilator dependency may be viewed by some professionals and laypersons as an unacceptable way of living, while others may feel that as long as there is life there is hope. The question thus arises: to whom is the quality of life unacceptable – is it the health-care staff, the patient, the patient's relatives or the community?

The ventilator-dependent patient is often viewed by health-care staff as the cause of futile and demanding work and the recipient of scarce resources that could be used to the benefit of someone else. The patient or the relatives may believe that as long as the patient is alive there is hope, and recovery is actually the hope that they may have been given when the patient was put on the ventilator in the first place. The patient's condition must be the subject of a consultative process involving the relatives, their advisors and the health-care team. The consultation should extend to explaining when there is a limitation on resources that will affect the care of the patient. It is essential to educate the relatives about the basis for the opinion that care is now futile, and to give them the opportunity to discuss and internalize the situation and to seek alternative opinions should they wish to do so. The passage of time is the greatest persuader that there will be no improvement in a patient's condition.

The community also has an interest in the ventilator-dependent patient, who is utilizing resources that are required to treat other patients in the community who may have better prospects of a favourable outcome.

Medication

Many medical staff, faced with life-threatening situations, will feel that they have to do *something*. They may institute therapy that is generally considered harmless and helpful, like antibiotics and cardiovascular support drugs, and give little consideration to the fact that some of these measures may have hidden harms to the patient, other patients and the institution as a whole. Apart from any risks of toxicity to already damaged organ systems, the latest antibiotics may cause resistant organisms to emerge, and these can be passed on to other patients. In addition, because the drugs are expensive, they may stretch the budget to the point that the institution cannot stock simple, cheap drugs. In contrast to decisions about surgery, decisions about the use of antibiotics and other drugs can seldom be shifted onto the patient or the patient's relatives. It would be unfair to ask relatives to bear the burden of decisions that involve shifting resources from others or to feel responsible for harm that might come to others.

The withdrawal of antibiotics, in a situation when care is considered futile, is intended to let sepsis take its course and is not obviously distressing to the patient. However, the decision should be discussed with the patient or relatives and the staff in case there is a legal challenge about the standard of treatment that has been given. The withdrawal of cardiovascular support drugs can be more dramatic, and the decision must be made openly if one is to avoid a possible legal challenge. Such decisions are best supported by institutional guidelines and protocols, along with mechanisms for discussing individual cases.

Food and water

Although withdrawal of ventilatory support or medications may hasten death, it may not, and discussions as well as court actions have centred around whether it is permissible to withhold water and nutrition in order to hasten death. There is a view that withdrawal of life-support measures in such cases amounts to euthanasia, and the expected effect of dehydration and starvation is repugnant to most health-care staff.

The courts have been petitioned against instituting such measures by doctors, relatives, institutions and community groups. Paradoxically, petitions to effect withdrawal usually come from patients' relatives when doctors and institutions have refused their requests to withdraw life-support measures. Obviously, decisions in these cases not only must be made with the support of staff but also should have the written informed consent of the next of kin.

The conscious patient

Withdrawal of life-support measures from a conscious patient may be perceived as euthanasia, even though that term is usually applied only to patients who are not considered to be dying. States of consciousness may vary, from an observer's perception of spontaneous eye-opening to the patient's explicit statement of being awake. When a patient is conscious enough to understand the issues and communicate, it is the patient, rather than relatives or staff, who should properly initiate any discussion on the matter of withdrawal of life-support measures. A judicial decision in *Wendland v. Wendland* provides guidance for occasions when the patient is conscious but has impaired understanding or communication: clear and convincing evidence of the patient's prior wishes is required to withdraw life-sustaining treatment in an impaired but conscious patient.

Decisions in court

Patients and their relatives faced with end-of-life decisions will often seek and rely on spiritual advice. When religious viewpoints conflict with professional advice, irreconcilable differences can be resolved only by the courts. It is hard for the courts to reconcile such opposing views in countries where there is a constitutional guarantee of religious freedom. However, the court is usually sympathetic to the medical professional's viewpoint on a life-and-death issue, particularly when it involves minors. For example, many might feel constrained to turn to the courts if faced with a young child (too young to be able to choose or understand the parents' religious views) with a bleeding disorder who is bleeding and requires blood products, and whose parents, being Jehovah's Witnesses, have refused to allow transfusion, which the doctors consider essential to saving the child's life. If the court agreed with the medical opinion, it would make the child a ward of the court and allow the treatment to proceed. Recourse to the courts is not normally pursued on behalf of adults or older children who are capable of making a choice, for the rights of all persons to hold their religious views as long as they are within the law should be respected [see Exercise 69].

Withdrawing life support

When life-support measures are withdrawn, the patient should not be abandoned. Every effort must be made to keep the patient comfortable and to have the support of family and spiritual counsellors. A problem with removing a ventilator, particularly from a conscious patient, is that the patient will experience discomfort as he or she struggles to breathe; this struggle can be relieved by the use of diazepam (Valium) and morphine, which makes the patient comfortable despite the fact that these drugs are known to cause respiratory depression.

The living will

The concept of the living will was introduced to give greater autonomy to the patient incapacitated by a terminal illness. Having considered the issue of life *per se* balanced against quality of life, many people seek to legally bind their next of kin and their physicians to a certain course of action in the event they become unable to participate in decisions about their care. Living wills are also intended to relieve physicians of the fear of legal liability should they, in carrying out a patient's wishes, appear to stray from the accepted standard of practice of the day. In reality, the doctor is being cast as a technical resource rather than as an advisor and protector of life, though in many cases the living will is drawn up with the full compliance of the doctor responsible for the patient's day-to-day care.

The person preparing a living will may specify a willingness to donate organs or may prescribe limits on the kind of medical interventions that he or she wishes to have in the event of a terminal illness that destroys their ability to make decisions. Living wills have to be carefully crafted legally to reflect a clear understanding of the possible illness.

Since there is no legal definition of dying, the question of when to activate the terms of a living will is inevitably open to interpretation. As for any other will, there has to be an executor, who might be the doctor or a relative; the executor, when faced with the reality of choosing life or death, particularly in an emergency situation, will often opt for life. As a result, living wills have not proven to be totally successful in preventing the institution of unwanted life-support measures and are seldom honoured in an emergency situation. In non-emergency situations, living wills may be resisted when they conflict with the moral or religious values of the staff who are asked to implement them.

Relatives, staff and the community may raise objections to the provisions of the living will and take the matter to court. For a living will to be effective, it must be drawn up with the willing consent of the responsible relative(s) and the physicians who will deal with the situation. If a doctor is presented with a living will and feels unable to carry out its requests, that should be conveyed to the patient or the patient's relatives and the institution's authorities (if applicable) right away.

The concept of a living will is quite separate from euthanasia: the latter is a conscious request for a medical practitioner to induce a person's death and contains no conditions related to the person's loss of control [see Exercise 70].

The right to die

The right to die in comfort and with dignity is a generally accepted standard in all communities and in all religions. Unfortunately, the prolonged use of modern life-support measures may leave the patient and the patient's relatives with a sense of discomfort and a loss of dignity, and may lead to a request for the removal of the life-support measures. If the professionals involved disagree with the removal of life-support measures, the patient or surrogate may petition the court.

Judges are not likely to side with the professional who argues for actions to prolong the process of dying. In several cases, courts have ruled to allow families to have ventilators withdrawn and, in some jurisdictions, artificial modes of hydration and nutrition stopped. The judge usually upholds the patient's right to autonomy; once convinced that withdrawal of life-support measures would have been the patient's wish, judges frequently grant the patient's relatives' request to allow the patient to die with dignity and without prolonging the process. However, where there is a chance of continued life, judges will err on the side of professional judgement. These considerations on the right to die are separate and distinct from the concept of euthanasia [see Exercise 71].

Euthanasia

A mentally or physically ill person who may not be dying but wishes to die faces the alternatives of committing suicide unaided or eliciting help in doing so. The latter is called euthanasia and, like suicide, is illegal in most jurisdictions. The role of the health-care team, when dealing with a patient who wishes to die, should be, first and foremost, to treat the patient's illness and try to dissuade the patient from suicide, either assisted or unassisted. Doctors, when they are aware of the risk of suicide, should not prescribe medication in such a quantity that the patient can succumb to the temptation to take an overdose. Admittedly, it is difficult to prevent patients from accumulating drugs or using non-prescription drugs or other means to commit suicide.

If a doctor actively renders medical treatment to cause the death of the patient at the patient's request, it is called euthanasia; however, the doctor can be charged before the court for murder. There are a few places in the world where euthanasia is legal or condoned. In the Netherlands thousands of cases of euthanasia occur each year. This situation came about after a doctor deliberately challenged the law and was tried and convicted, but the authorities said that in future euthanasia could be practised under certain conditions. These conditions specified that the patient must have made a clear declaration of intent when he or she was capable of making the decision, that the doctor must obtain the consenting opinion of another practitioner, and that the event should be reported to the police, who agreed not to prosecute under those circumstances. However, euthanasia remained "illegal" for another 20 years before the law was changed.

Modern ethical practice stresses the right of people to make decisions about the fate of their bodies. For the medical practitioner, however, the ethical acceptability of euthanasia presents a quandary, for it is always difficult to rationalize going against the imperative of "thou shall not kill", particularly when the individual is not a threat to society. The challenge for the community in accepting the practice of euthanasia is to ensure that the ill, the old and the disabled will not be made to feel that they are a burden to the society and as a result request euthanasia [see Exercise 23].

The use of narcotic analgesia

Disputes about the proper treatment and relief of pain and suffering are frequent in the treatment of the terminally ill. Most of the contention arises over narcotic analgesia, for while narcotics are excellent pain relievers they may also cause respiratory depression and hasten death. There is also an unworthy contention that narcotics may cause addiction in the terminally ill patient. Ambivalence over these issues has been compounded by the fact that narcotics have been used by health-care professionals to commit euthanasia and murder.

The risks and benefits of narcotic analgesia, as for any other treatment, should be explained to the patient and the patient's relatives, and a conscious choice should be made either to use or not to use them. When used, they should be given in sufficient quantity and frequency to relieve the pain, with full knowledge of the likely but unintended respiratory complication [see Exercise 72].

The role of ethicists and ethical committees

The role of an ethicist or an ethical committee in resolving conflicting viewpoints must be different from that of the court. A judge is asked to make a binding decision between the positions of contending parties. A committee can be a sounding board which does not decide for one or the other side but enables both sides to be heard and other viewpoints and experiences to be brought forward for the consideration of both sides. Thus, patients and their surrogates might hear other religious viewpoints on the sanctity of life and how there are times when such ultimate choices may have to be made by a court.

Doctors may need to be reminded of the rights and autonomy of patients, parents and guardians, and of the need to respect their religious views. They might also be asked questions such as whether their insistence on a course of action is prejudiced by the technological challenge or by the nationality, social status or ethnicity of the patient. Where religious viewpoints are prominent, doctors may need to be asked whether their decision to challenge the patient would have been different if they shared the patient's religious convictions.

These are questions that a committee can ask without having to decide for one viewpoint or the other, but which could make the contending parties think through their decisions with greater clarity. As discussion and exploration of the issues goes on, decisions often become obvious [see Exercise 73].

Exercises 60 to 73

The following scenarios are based on events in practice. Identify the ethical and legal issues and state whether the conduct of the professionals was correct and why. If the professional conduct was not correct, state what it should have been. Discussion follows the exercises.

◆ Exercise 60

A mother brings her 14-year-old daughter to see a gynaecologist and says that the girl has missed her menstrual periods. The mother says she thinks her daughter is pregnant and wants her to have an abortion. The doctor examines the girl, confirms that she is pregnant and tells the mother that abortion is against the law. The mother retorts, "But she was raped!" The doctor responds that the law does not allow it even for rape. The mother says, "You want me to take her into some back street? Don't you know anyone here or abroad who will do it properly?"

◆ Exercise 61

The staff of an *in vitro* fertilization clinic have organized a "reunion" of families to celebrate the clinic's twentieth anniversary. A book has been prepared for the occasion, and at the reunion one of the clients remarks that a number of the children look like brothers and sisters. When a group photograph is being taken of Dr Ego and the children, the impression is reinforced, and Mr Law says to his wife, "Don't you think that most of the children look like the doctor?"

◆ Exercise 62

Mr and Mrs Furtole have been unable to have children. Their doctor has recommended that an ovum from another woman be fertilized with the husband's sperm and implanted into the wife's womb. The couple are given the profiles of several women, and after choosing, they are given a contract to sign in which they agree to pay for the medical and personal services of the ovum donor. Mrs Furtole asks if she can meet the woman. The doctor replies that this is not encouraged but if the Furtoles insist, she will ask the young woman if she wishes to meet with them.

◆ Exercise 63

Dr Furlonge runs a very busy and successful *in vitro* fertilization clinic, serving clients from many different parts of the country and even from abroad. As often happens, he receives a letter from one his clients when the baby is successfully born. This letter includes a photograph of the couple with their baby. The husband writes that he will probably be the butt of jokes at the office – his mates will say that not only couldn't he make it but he allowed his wife to choose a white man's sperm. He goes on to say that he is happy and that he will tell his mates that the child is a throwback to when the slave master impregnated his great-great-grandmother. Dr Furlonge is a little puzzled, checks his records and finds that the couple had used the husband's sperm. About a week later, he receives a letter and a photograph from another couple, who say they are really excited about their child, but they are being asked why the child is so dark. "We tell everyone, 'That's exactly what we asked for – it's time to integrate the neighbourhood!' Well, my husband thinks that you may have mixed up his sperm with someone else's, but I tell him that can't happen with all the precautions your assistant showed us. Anyway he so loves the baby that he is already talking about getting another."

◆ Exercise 64

The Despers have been childless, and their hopes seem to have come to an end because Mrs Desper has had to have a hysterectomy. They are thinking about adoption when one of their employees says, "Why don't you get somebody to carry the pregnancy for you? I wouldn't mind doing it." They arrange a consultation at the clinic, and a contract is drawn up specifying that the Despers will pay all the medical expenses plus a fee of $20,000 and the surrogate mother will keep her job at the firm as long as she wishes. A fertilized ovum from the Despers is successfully implanted, and nine months later the child is born. Two days after delivery, the surrogate mother says she wants to change the contract before she gives up the baby – she would like to be recognized as the mother should anything happen to the Despers.

◆ Exercise 65

Dr Brash has run a successful *in vitro* fertilization clinic for the past 25 years. At a staff meeting, the question arises of whether they should explore the techniques of cloning and offer it as a service. After discussion, Dr Brash says that although it is a controversial area she feels that it should be explored, and when they are ready she will not only take the heat but also be the first to have it done.

◆ Exercise 66

Following an uneventful pregnancy, Mrs Dervoute has had a prolonged and difficult labour. After performing several procedures, the obstetrician has decided that the labour is obstructed and, after consulting with a senior colleague, has told the

Dervoutes that the best solution is to abort the baby. Mr Dervoute responds that they cannot accept that and asks if there is not another way. One of the obstetricians says that there is an old procedure of splitting the pelvis but he doubts, given Mrs Dervoute's condition, that either mother or baby will survive. Mr Dervoute says, "That is what you will have to do, and at least my soul and theirs may be able to rest in peace."

◆ Exercise 67

Mrs Pretticote has had an ultrasound examination of her pregnancy and is told that her child has a congenital defect in its abdomen which will need to be operated on when the child is born. In response to her questions, she is told that the child will probably be normal after the operation. She returns to the clinic shortly thereafter and says that, having thought about it, she would like to have the foetus aborted. The doctor counsels her that there is no need to abort the infant because of this kind of abnormality, but Mrs Pretticote insists that this is what she wants done.

◆ Exercise 68

A 75-year-old known hypertensive man is admitted with a cerebrovascular accident (CVA), deeply unconscious and with difficulty breathing. He is placed on a ventilator. A CT scan is done which shows an intracerebral haemorrhage involving the brain stem. After four days, Dr Driver, the head of the unit, extubates the patient, declaring that he is brain-dead, and asks that the ventilator be prepared for a patient to be admitted from the accident and emergency department. An hour later, Mr Driver, who was involved in a road traffic accident and has a head injury, is admitted and placed on the ventilator.

◆ Exercise 69

Mr Carless suffered a severe head injury in a road accident and has been on a ventilator for two months without any improvement in his condition: he is in a coma and in a decerebrate posture. Dr Logic speaks to Mr Carless's parents, telling them that their son is not going to recover and recommending that he be removed from the ventilator. The parents respond that they have been praying every day, and that the priest tells them to hang on because "you never know when a miracle will occur". Dr Logic responds that he doesn't believe in miracles and asks them if they would like a second opinion.

◆ Exercise 70

Mrs Curtis's father, brother and sister all died suddenly from ruptured intracerebral aneurysms. After speaking to her doctor, Mrs Curtis has her lawyer draw up a living will stating that if a similar thing happens to her she does not want to be put on a ventilator. She is found unconscious at home by a neighbour, who calls an emergency ambulance. As she is being taken away by the ambulance attendants, the neighbour says to them, "The same thing happened to her father, brother and sister, and she signed a paper saying that she does not want to be put on any machines." After she arrives at the hospital, a provisional diagnosis is made of a ruptured intracerebral aneurysm, and she is put on a ventilator.

◆ Exercise 71

Mr Curtis has returned from overseas to see his mother, who has been admitted to hospital and is on a ventilator with a diagnosis of a ruptured intracerebral aneurysm. He recalls his mother saying that before his uncle and aunt died they had been kept on ventilators for a long time, and that she did not want to die like that. He asks to see the doctors, and after discussing her condition, he asks that his mother be removed from the ventilator so that she can die in peace. The doctors refuse to do so since removal of the ventilator will result in her death, and it is against hospital policy to remove anyone from a ventilator before death.

◆ Exercise 72

An 86-year-old woman has a disseminated carcinoma and is in severe pain. Her son, who has been praying with her every day, asks the nurse if his mother may have some more medication. The nurse responds that she has had what was prescribed and if she gets more "it could produce complications". The son then meets the doctor on the corridor and asks the same question. The doctor says that he will give her morphine but that she may not be able to talk with her son as much, and she will probably die sooner.

◆ Exercise 73

A surgeon is asked to see a newborn with a large swelling in the upper thigh. A sarcoma is diagnosed, and the surgeon advises the parents that the best treatment is to remove the tumour and follow up with chemotherapy. The parents tell the doctor to do what is best but specify that the child should not get a blood transfusion. The surgeon responds that to do the operation without a blood transfusion would be dangerous, and he could not agree to do it; he then asks whether they would like to get another opinion. After the second opinion confirms that operation is the best course, the parents insist that the surgeon should operate on the child without the use of blood.

Discussion

The following discussions address the issues of professional conduct raised in the exercises. Other conclusions are possible.

Exercise 60

Issues

- What is the law regarding abortion in the jurisdiction?
- Should the doctor adhere to the law under all circumstances?
- Should the doctor refer to others who will act outside of the law?

Professional conduct

- Health professionals should know the law in the area in which they practise. If they are not familiar with all of the limitations of the law, they should seek advice from knowledgeable colleagues, institutional resources, professional organizations or their professional liability company.
- Health professionals should always adhere to the law in the jurisdiction where they practise. However, changes in the law have come about as a result of some physicians' carrying out acts of civil disobedience and courting prosecution but, in doing so, bringing to public attention what they consider unjust laws. This course cannot be recommended by a body of professionals, although it may be carried out by individuals prepared to make sacrifices.
- Professionals should not refer patients to unqualified persons or to those who they know will break the law. However, if different laws and practice obtain in another jurisdiction, the patient can be referred to a professional in that jurisdiction, providing no other laws are contravened.

Exercise 61

Issues

- Are there any ethical or legal implications in a reunion of this sort?
- The suspicion is raised that the doctor has been the sperm donor in a number of the cases. Is there anything wrong with that?

Professional conduct

- There is the issue of breaching confidentiality of the families. This potential problem could be overcome if all families were made aware of the implications of attending such an event, which might attract wider publicity; then only those explicitly willing to take the risk would attend. There could also be a breach of confidentiality if any family who did not wish to take part was referred to in any way in the reunion book or events.

- It is unwise of staff who deal with sensitive anonymous situations to offer or impose themselves as genetic donors for their clients. The discovery of any unwanted genetic trait could lead to an accusation of battery on grounds of deliberately producing harm without truly informed consent.

◆ Exercise 62

Issues

- Is it legal to buy living tissue from another human being?
- Should donors of genetic material remain anonymous to the recipient?
- Why should the meeting of a genetic donor and the recipient be discouraged?

Professional conduct

- The legality of such transactions varies between jurisdictions, and within a particular jurisdiction it may vary depending on the kind of tissue being purchased. For example, it may be legal to purchase blood, an ovum or sperm but illegal to purchase organs for transplantation, as generally obtains in the United States. In other countries, the purchase of blood is not allowed, although blood products are sold; elsewhere ova and sperm may be bought only indirectly; and in some countries organs may be purchased.
- In general, the purchase of human materials tends to exploit the poor, who seek to donate for economic gain and who may not be made aware of the risks involved, even when they are significant, as the purchaser seeks to obtain scarce material. Purchase rather than donation also carries a risk of transmission of disease – both infections and genetic disorders – to the recipient. With the donation of sperm, the risks are primarily to the recipient, whereas with the donation of ova there are significant risks to the donor related to the medical and surgical procedures to be done.
- Genes contribute to a person's physical development, disease processes and probably psychological make-up. Children become curious about their genetic parents when a situation arises that leads them to suspect that their legal parents are not their genetic parents. Except in the case of relatives, the donors themselves may not wish to accept the responsibility of being claimed as a parent by the child. It is therefore prudent to keep the donor's identity anonymous, although the donor's physical characteristics and personal and family medical history should be known to the prospective legal parents.

- In spite of the information given about the donor, a recipient may still have doubts which might be resolved by a face-to-face encounter. Such encounters cannot be guaranteed to resolve all doubts about the donor, and certainly are unlikely to enable the recipient to accurately predict the characteristics of the potential child. They are also unfair to the donor, who usually enters into the "contract" with the expectation that personal scrutiny will not be required and that he or she will be shielded from the emotional responsibility of knowing the child that carries the donor's genes.

◆ Exercise 63

Issues

- The circumstances suggest that there has been a switch of genetic material. How should the doctor respond?
- The couples seem happy with their babies; should the doubts be investigated?

Professional conduct

- Dr Furlonge must seek the truth and reveal it in an appropriate way. To that end, a detailed internal investigation should be carried out to see whether a switch of genetic material could have been made at any stage. The temporal proximity of the two letters suggests that a switch could have occurred when the embryos were implanted. The internal analysis should include the DNA analysis of any sperm or embryos that have been preserved.
- Although the letters do not suggest that any action is contemplated against the doctor and the clinic, there is every possibility that, at some time, DNA analyses may be done on the infants and it will be discovered that they do not carry their parents' genetic imprint. Dr Furlonge would therefore be wise to seek, as sensitively as possible, to obtain DNA samples from both children and compare them with the genetic material of the parents. There is no need initially for the doctor to reveal his suspicions to the individual couples.
- If the suspicions are confirmed, the couples should be counselled separately to determine if there is any desire to exchange infants. If the desire exists on both sides, a switch can be effected. If there is a desire not to switch on one or both sides, the doctor should seek legal advice and the advice of counsellors to determine whether the couples should be identified to each other.

◆ Exercise 64

Issues

- Is there a legal distinction between a birth mother and a genetic mother?
- Can a legitimate contract be made to buy or sell a child?
- Can a surrogate contract be enforced if the birth mother or the genetic parents change their minds?

Professional conduct

- A mother is recognized in law by having given birth to the child or by obtaining legal guardianship through adoption. There is no legal claim to a child on the basis of a genetic imprint alone, unless a specific statute has been passed in the jurisdiction, and such a claim would have to be decided in court.
- The purchase of a child is generally against the law in most jurisdictions; however, most jurisdictions allow for reimbursement of expenses incurred to surrogate mothers. The law varies among jurisdictions as to whether a surrogacy contract is enforceable in law, and in some jurisdictions making arrangements for any form of payment is an offence.
- The enforcement of a contract will depend on whether the contract was considered legal in the jurisdiction. In the absence of specific statutes, most jurisdictions would make a decision that is considered in the best interest of the child, giving due weight to the conventional rights of the birth mother.

◆ Exercise 65

Issues

- What are the motives for cloning?
- Is cloning a human being legal?
- Do clones develop normally?
- What are the views of organized religion on cloning?
- What are the relationships of a clone to the family and the community?
- Can clones be used as a spare-organ "factory"?

Professional conduct

- The obvious motive for cloning oneself is love of self; the motive for cloning another person would be to reproduce some admired quality in another. The decision to clone presupposes that a near-perfect reproduction will be achieved without any significant influence of the intrauterine or extrauterine environment.
- There is no natural or other law that anticipates the possibility of cloning. In most

communities the developmental abnormalities that emerge from close-family reproduction – for example, among siblings – have been observed, and in many places marriage between close relatives has been forbidden in law. Reproductive technologies have tended to outstrip the legislative response to the ethical and legal issues raised by those technologies, and there are only a few jurisdictions that address the issues of cloning by banning it; otherwise, it is assumed to be legal where the law is silent.

- The limited experience in animal cloning has shown so far that cloned embryos are likely to have developmental abnormalities. Those few embryos that have developed normally have shown signs of premature aging. There is no good information as yet on the behavioural characteristics of cloned animals. If behavioural characteristics turn out to be the same, will they evolve at the pace of normal human growth, or will the cloned child have the behaviour of a normal adult?

- There is nothing in the traditional religions' texts or teachings that anticipates cloning, and most religious leaders tend not to favour it. One religious sect, the Raelians, teaches that humans are cloned from aliens who came to Earth from outer space.

- Clones would redefine the whole basis of family relationships, in that it could be argued that a clone was at once a sibling and a child of the genetic donor. With the increasing use of genetic markers in the community, it would not be possible to determine identity by the DNA fingerprint in either criminal proceedings or paternity/maternity issues.

- Perhaps the most repulsive possibility is that a clone could be developed to provide an organ bank for the purpose of prolonging life and even achieving the dream of "everlasting" life. Man has shown the capacity to follow his imagination, and this possibility cannot be dismissed.

◆ Exercise 66

Issues

- Should the husband be making such decisions related to his wife's life?
- Should the doctors accept the decision to risk the mother's life to save the child?
- Can the doctors challenge the husband's decision?

Professional conduct

- In most jurisdictions, decisions about treatment are for the competent patient to make. In some jurisdictions, however, particularly those ruled by Islamic law, a husband has the legal power to make decisions about his wife's treatment. In situations such as that described, the woman may be too ill or too sedated to make the decision, and the husband is the legally competent person to do so.

- Fathers, whether they are husbands or not, have a right to take part in decisions about the care of their child, and if the views differ between father and mother and cannot be reconciled, only the court can settle the matter.
- When patients or their surrogates disagree with the doctor's advice, second opinions should be offered, as well as ethical – and, where appropriate, legal – advice. Doctors have an overriding duty to preserve life. When a conflict arises between one life and another, a number of factors must be taken into account, particularly that of who has the best chance of survival with a good quality of life.
- In the case described, it appears that religious considerations may be the overriding factor in the husband's decision. While these views should be respected, if they endanger a life that could be saved, the doctor may appeal to the court to overturn the decision of the surrogate decision-maker. Doctors should be reluctant to challenge a similar decision made by the mother herself.

◆ Exercise 67

Issues

- What is the purpose of diagnosing foetal abnormalities before birth?
- Should the doctor heed the patient's wishes?

Professional conduct

- The purpose of any investigation should be made known to the patient, and the patient should understand what the consequences of the results will be. It appears as if this doctor and patient may have had in mind different reasons for the investigation. The doctor may well have wished to have as much information as possible to plan for treatment; the patient may well have understood the investigation to be done to ensure that all was normal with the pregnancy.
- The doctor appears to be caught in a dilemma: he has diagnosed an abnormal foetus, but the patient is not prepared to accept the doctor's opinion that the abnormality can be remedied. The patient appears to have decided that an abnormal foetus should be aborted, and such a view may be difficult to change unless the issue has been discussed previously. It is important to counsel patients before carrying out investigations that may reveal sensitive diagnoses requiring difficult decisions.
- If the doctor does not agree with a course of treatment that a patient wishes to pursue, he or she can refuse to treat the patient. In refusing to treat, a doctor must be aware that the patient may seek alternatives which may not be in the patient's best interest. In some circumstances, if the doctor is refusing to treat because of a

conscientious objection, he or she should suggest another professional to see the patient.

◆ Exercise 68

Issues

- Is it futile treatment to place an elderly patient with a CVA on a ventilator?
- Has the doctor made the diagnosis of brain death in the appropriate manner?
- Can the doctor simply stop ventilation on a brain-dead patient?
- Is there some impropriety in removing a patient from life support to place another patient on such support?

Professional conduct

- Although it may appear futile to have placed an elderly patient with a diagnosed CVA on a ventilator, there may have been some uncertainty about the prospect of recovery until further investigation was done. Doctors may also have responded to the emergency situation of difficulty in breathing and diagnosed the CVA only after ventilatory support was established. Once the conclusion has been reached that therapy is futile, then the criterion on which the decision was made, such as brain death, should be conveyed to the relatives and the staff, and discussion about cessation of the futile therapy should be initiated.

- Depending on the jurisdiction, the diagnosis of brain death may be made on clinical criteria alone or backed up with confirmatory evidence of a lack of brain activity or cerebral circulation. The determination should be made by at least two physicians, one of whom is preferably a neurologist, and the findings documented in the notes. The circumstance described does not suggest that standard procedure, including independent confirmation, has been followed.

- In jurisdictions where brain death is an established legal diagnosis, the physician is entitled to cease treatment as for any other dead person. However, relatives and other caregivers may not have internalized the diagnosis, and the removal of a ventilator, causing the more conventional and accepted death, could be misinterpreted. In making the diagnosis of brain death, it is prudent to be transparent to all and to make sure relatives and staff know why the diagnosis is being made – whether to facilitate organ donation or to release resources for the treatment of others.

- In the case described, withdrawal of ventilation appears to facilitate the use of the ventilator for a patient who may be a relative of the doctor making the decision. Such a situation may well draw a charge of impropriety; the diagnosis should be clearly documented, and the decision confirmed by an independent physician.

◆ Exercise 69

Issues

- What is the anticipated effect of removing the ventilator?
- Do the parents have any say in deciding whether treatment should be discontinued?
- What should the doctor do if the ventilator is required for someone else?

Professional conduct

- The patient in a persistent vegetative state should be able to breathe spontaneously and may live, with other supportive measures, without a ventilator. Ventilation may therefore be seen as futile treatment, in the sense that it will not improve the patient's condition, and consideration should be given to its being withdrawn.
- Parents, as the surrogate decision makers, do have a role in consenting to what treatment should be carried out. However, the parents have no role in deciding what treatment should be carried out or withdrawn. If withdrawing treatment could be shown to cause harm to the patient, the parents could appeal to the courts if the doctor decided to withdraw treatment in spite of their objections.
- The doctor may have a responsibility to treat more than one patient, and resources may be limited. If ventilation treatment is futile or ineffective for one patient, and the resource is needed for another patient who has a chance of recovery, then the doctor has a responsibility to mobilize the resources to treat the patient who may benefit. This should be done in full consultation with both family and the staff treating the patient from whom the resource is being withdrawn, and preferably with an independent second opinion so that the reallocation of the resource is not misunderstood.

◆ Exercise 70

Issues

- Has the living will been properly formulated?
- Have the doctors acted improperly or illegally by acting against the patient's wishes?

Professional conduct

- The patient has attempted to control how she would wish to be treated, following the advice of the professional she has consulted on the matter. She has also made her wishes known, so that her neighbour is also familiar with her wishes and attempts to convey those wishes to the caregivers. Nevertheless, her wishes were not adhered to.

- In most emergency situations, the physicians involved would not have had prior knowledge of a living-will provision, and it would be imprudent for them to rely on hearsay; they should therefore carry out the normal standard of care. When the provisions of a living will have been confirmed, the physicians in charge should discuss the provisions with the responsible next of kin and decide whether to adhere to the provisions of the will by not instituting treatment or by reversing what may have been started.

◆ Exercise 71

Issues

- What role does a patient's son have in making decisions about his mother's care?
- Should the doctors entertain the request from a surrogate to stop life support?
- Can the hospital make policies to direct a doctor's actions?
- What recourse does the son have in relation to the refusal of his request?

Professional conduct

- When a patient is incapacitated and unable to make decisions about treatment, those decisions are legally made by the next of kin or other guardian – for example, the head of an institution if the patient has been institutionalized. A child who has reached the age of majority may be the next of kin and therefore has the capacity to consent to or refuse treatment on behalf of the patient.
- Doctors must consider the legally competent person responsible for consenting to treatment as also being able to refuse treatment. Should the doctors wish to go against the surrogate's wishes, they should do so on the grounds that to comply with the surrogate's wishes would be unlawful, and they should either seek legal advice on the matter or request to be released from the care of the patient.
- Hospitals should have policies in place for the guidance of staff. Mechanisms should include ethical and legal advice to deal with situations of conflict. Where there are irreconcilable differences between the institution and a patient's surrogate, the institution may wish to obtain guidance from the court.
- The son, as the responsible surrogate, can petition the court to direct the doctors and the hospital to carry out his wishes to have his mother removed from the ventilator. The court will hear expert testimony on the prospects of the patient's recovery, as well as testimony and any documentary evidence regarding the wishes that the patient would have had on the matter. It is likely, in the circumstances described, that the court will find against the doctors and the hospital.

◆ Exercise 72

Issues

- Are the nurses and doctors managing this patient's situation properly?
- Should medications that hasten death be given?

Professional conduct

- There appears to be little communication between the staff and the patient herself about the degree of her pain, how it can best be relieved and the possible drawbacks of the available medications.
- The nurse has responded to the enquiry with facts about the medication but has offered no help, such as asking the doctor to review the situation with the patient or the enquiring relative.
- The doctor has promised to give the patient another drug and has told the relative what the complications may be; however, the doctor has not indicated that any attempt will be made to discuss the situation with the patient in order to discern her wishes.

◆ Exercise 73

Issues

- Should the surgeon do the operation against his or her best judgement?
- Are there other consultations that should be offered to the parents?
- Can the parents' wishes be countermanded?

Professional conduct

- The surgeon has properly given an opinion and refused to operate under circumstances which, in his or her judgement, may cause harm. The offer of a second opinion about the suggested treatment has been given, but the question of the need or otherwise for blood transfusion does not appear to have been addressed.
- The parents apparently require more information or opinions about the need for blood transfusion and may benefit from discussions with others who are uninvolved in the proposed surgery. Discussion with an ethical committee may help them understand the stance taken by the surgeon; they may believe that the surgeon is simply reacting against their religious viewpoint.
- In discussions with the parents, it could be explained to them that if they are thought to be endangering the life of their child, the doctors could petition to have the child designated a ward of the court, which would then decide what treatment

should be followed. Such a petition should not be undertaken before exploring all other avenues of persuasion. In the case described, the petition should be entertained only if the doctors are convinced that the child has a high probability of being cured and that the treatment they propose is indeed the only course to be followed.

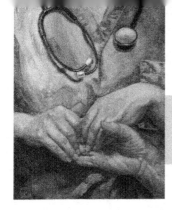

CHAPTER 9

Research Ethics

Improving the quality of health care depends on the examination of outcomes and the introduction of new or improved medications and procedures that are intended to produce better outcomes. Determining the value of a new drug or procedure requires a search for the truth, and research is the way we examine the probability that the answer is true. Since answers to human reactions cannot all be determined in the laboratory or through animal experimentation, experimentation with humans is a vital part of the quest for improved outcomes in health care. Research involving human beings requires the strict observance of the ethical principles of beneficence, non-malfeasance, autonomy and justice. This is particularly important because the outcomes are unknown, although the analysis of previous studies and work in the laboratory or on animals may have demonstrated the safety of the proposed intervention in similar circumstances.

Unfortunately, in the quest for new knowledge, some researchers have ignored ethical principles. The most notorious such lapses in modern history became public during the war crime trials after World War II. As a result of those trials, which were held at Nuremberg, Germany, the code reproduced here (Figure 5) was formulated (Connor and Fuenzalida-Puelma 1990, 217–18). In spite of undergoing many refinements since they were formulated, the principles enunciated in the code still stand as the guide to the ethical conduct of research. Further refinements to the code and guidelines for research have been worked out under the aegis of the International Organization of Medical Sciences, the World Health Organization and the World Medical Association, which produced the widely used Declaration of Helsinki (Figure 6) (Connor and Fuenzalida-Puelma 1990, 218–20).

Figure 5

The Nuremberg Code

International Tribunal of Nuremberg, 1947

Permitted Medical Experiments

The great weight of the evidence before us is to the effect that certain types of medical experiments on human beings, when kept within reasonably well-defined bounds, conform to the ethics of the medical profession generally. The protagonists of the practice of human experimentation justify their views on the basis that such experiments yield results for the good of society that are unprocurable by other methods or means of study. All agree, however, that certain basic principles must be observed in order to satisfy moral, ethical, and legal concepts:

1. The voluntary consent of the human subject is absolutely essential. This means that the person involved should have legal capacity to give consent; should be so situated as to be able to exercise free power of choice, without the intervention of any element of force, fraud, deceit, duress, overreaching, or other ulterior form of constraint or coercion; and should have sufficient knowledge and comprehension of the elements of the subject matter involved as to enable him to make an understanding and enlightened decision. This latter element requires that before the acceptance of an affirmative decision by the experimental subject there should be made known to him the nature, duration, and purpose of the experiment; the method and means by which it is to be conducted; any inconveniences and hazards reasonably to be expected; and the effects upon his health or person which may possibly come from his participation in the experiment.

    The duty and responsibility for ascertaining the quality of the consent rests upon each individual who initiates, directs, or engages in the experiment. It is a personal duty and responsibility which may not be delegated to another with impunity.

2. The experiment should be such as to yield fruitful results for the good of society, unprocurable by other methods or means of study, and not random and unnecessary in nature.

3. The experiment should be so designed and based on the results of animal experimentation and a knowledge of the natural history of the disease or other problem under study that the anticipated results will justify the performance of the experiment.

4. The experiment should be so conducted as to avoid all unnecessary physical and mental suffering and injury.

5. No experiment should be conducted where there is an a priori reason to believe that death or disabling injury will occur; except, perhaps, in those experiments where the experimental physicians also serve as subjects.

6. The degree of risk to be taken should never exceed that determined by the humanitarian importance of the problem to be solved by the experiment.

Figure 5 continues

Figure 5

7. Proper preparations should be made and adequate facilities provided to protect the experimental subject against even remote possibilities of injury, disability, or death.
8. The experiment should be conducted only by scientifically qualified persons. The highest degree of skill and care should be required through all stages of the experiment of those who conduct or engage in the experiment.
9. During the course of the experiment the human subject should be at liberty to bring the experiment to an end if he has reached the physical or mental state where continuation of the experiment seems to him to be impossible.
10. During the course of the experiment the scientist in charge must be prepared to terminate the experiment at any stage, if he has probable cause to believe, in the exercise of the good faith, superior skill, and careful judgment required of him, that a continuation of the experiment is likely to result in injury, disability, or death to the experimental subject.

Figure 6

World Medical Association Declaration of Helsinki
Ethical Principles for Medical Research Involving Human Subjects

Adopted by the 18th WMA General Assembly, Helsinki, Finland, June 1964, and amended by the 29th WMA General Assembly, Tokyo, Japan, October 1975, the 35th WMA General Assembly, Venice, Italy, October 1983, the 41st WMA General Assembly, Hong Kong, September 1989, the 48th WMA General Assembly, Somerset West, Republic of South Africa, October 1996, and the 52nd WMA General Assembly, Edinburgh, Scotland, October 2000

A. Introduction

1. The World Medical Association has developed the Declaration of Helsinki as a statement of ethical principles to provide guidance to physicians and other participants in medical research involving human subjects. Medical research involving human subjects includes research on identifiable human material or identifiable data.
2. It is the duty of the physician to promote and safeguard the health of the people. The physician's knowledge and conscience are dedicated to the fulfilment of this duty.
3. The Declaration of Geneva of the World Medical Association binds the physician with the words, "The health of my patient will be my first consideration," and the International Code of Medical Ethics declares that, "A Physician shall act only in the patient's interest when providing medical care which might have the effect of weakening the physical and mental condition of the patient."
4. Medical progress is based on research which ultimately must rest in part on experimentation involving human subjects.
5. In medical research on human subjects, considerations related to the well-being of the human subject should take precedence over the interests of science and society.

Figure 6 continues

Figure 6

6. The primary purpose of medical research involving human subjects is to improve prophylactic, diagnostic and therapeutic procedures and the understanding of the aetiology and pathogenesis of disease. Even the best proven prophylactic, diagnostic, and therapeutic methods must continuously be challenged through research for their effectiveness, efficiency, accessibility and quality.

7. In current medical practice and in medical research, most prophylactic, diagnostic and therapeutic procedures involve risks and burdens.

8. Medical research is subject to ethical standards that promote respect for all human beings and protect their health and rights. Some research populations are vulnerable and need special protection. The particular needs of the economically and medically disadvantaged must be recognized. Special attention is also required for those who cannot give or refuse consent for themselves, for those who may be subject to giving consent under duress, for those who will not benefit personally from the research and for those for whom the research is combined with care.

9. Research Investigators should be aware of the ethical, legal and regulatory requirements; for research on human subjects in their own countries as well as applicable international requirements. No national ethical, legal or regulatory requirement should be allowed to reduce or eliminate any of the protections for human subjects set forth in this Declaration.

B. Basic Principles for all Medical Research

10. It is the duty of the physician in medical research to protect the life, health, privacy, and dignity of the human subject.

11. Medical research involving human subjects must conform to generally accepted scientific principles, be based on a thorough knowledge of the scientific literature, other relevant sources of information, and on adequate laboratory and, where appropriate, animal experimentation.

12. Appropriate caution must be exercised in the conduct of research which may affect the environment, and the welfare of animals used for research must be respected.

13. The design and performance of each experimental procedure involving human subjects should be clearly formulated in an experimental protocol. This protocol should be submitted for consideration, comment, guidance, and where appropriate, approval to a specially appointed ethical review committee, which must be independent of the investigator, the sponsor or any other kind of undue influence. This independent committee should be in conformity with the laws and regulations of the country in which the research experiment is performed. The committee has the right to monitor ongoing trials. The researcher has the obligation to provide monitoring information to the committee, especially any serious adverse events. The researcher should also submit to the committee, for review, information regarding funding, sponsors, institutional affiliations, other potential conflicts of interest and incentives for subjects.

14. The research protocol should always contain a statement of the ethical considerations involved and should indicate that there is compliance with the principles enunciated in this Declaration.

Figure 6 continues

Figure 6

15. Medical research involving human subjects should be conducted only by scientifically qualified persons and under the supervision of a clinically competent medical person. The responsibility for the human subject must always rest with a medically qualified person and never rest on the subject of the research, even though the subject has given consent.

16. Every medical research project involving human subjects should be preceded by careful assessment of predictable risks and burdens in comparison with foreseeable benefits to the subject or to others. This does not preclude the participation of healthy volunteers in medical research. The design of all studies should be publicly available.

17. Physicians should abstain from engaging in research projects involving human subjects unless they are confident that the risks involved have been adequately assessed and can be satisfactorily managed. Physicians should cease any investigation if the risks are found to outweigh the potential benefits or if there is conclusive proof of positive and beneficial results.

18. Medical research involving human subjects should only be conducted if the importance of the objective outweighs the inherent risks and burdens to the subject. This is especially important when the human subjects are healthy volunteers.

19. Medical research is only justified if there is a reasonable likelihood that the populations in which the research is carried out stand to benefit from the results of the research.

20. The subjects must be volunteers and informed participants in the research project.

21. The right of research subjects to safeguard their integrity must always be respected. Every precaution should be taken to respect the privacy of the subject, the confidentiality of the patient's information and to minimize the impact of the study on the subject's physical and mental integrity and on the personality of the subject.

22. In any research on human beings, each potential subject must be adequately informed of the aims, methods, sources of funding, any possible conflicts of interest, institutional affiliations of the researcher, the anticipated benefits and potential risks of the study and the discomfort it may entail. The subject should be informed of the right to abstain from participation in the study or to withdraw consent to participate at any time without reprisal. After ensuring that the subject has understood the information, the physician should then obtain the subject's freely given informed consent, preferably in writing. If the consent cannot be obtained in writing, the non-written consent must be formally documented and witnessed.

23. When obtaining informed consent for the research project the physician should be particularly cautious if the subject is in a dependent relationship with the physician or may consent under duress. In that case the informed consent should be obtained by a well-informed physician who is not engaged in the investigation and who is completely independent of this relationship.

24. For a research subject who is legally incompetent, physically or mentally incapable of giving consent or is a legally incompetent minor, the investigator must obtain informed consent from the legally authorized representative in accordance with applicable law.

Figure 6 continues

Figure 6

These groups should not be included in research unless the research is necessary to promote the health of the population represented and this research cannot instead be performed on legally competent persons.

25. When a subject deemed legally incompetent, such as a minor child, is able to give assent to decisions about participation in research, the investigator must obtain that assent in addition to the consent of the legally authorized representative.

26. Research on individuals from whom it is not possible to obtain consent, including proxy or advance consent, should be done only if the physical/mental condition that prevents obtaining informed consent is a necessary characteristic of the research population. The specific reasons for involving research subjects with a condition that renders them unable to give informed consent should be stated in the experimental protocol for consideration and approval of the review committee. The protocol should state that consent to remain in the research should be obtained as soon as possible from the individual or a legally authorized surrogate.

27. Both authors and publishers have ethical obligations. In publication of the results of research, the investigators are obliged to preserve the accuracy of the results. Negative as well as positive results should be published or otherwise publicly available. Sources of funding, institutional affiliations and any possible conflicts of interest should be declared in the publication. Reports of experimentation not in accordance with the principles laid down in this Declaration should not be accepted for publication.

C. Additional Principles for Medical Research Combined with Medical Care

28. The physician may combine medical research with medical care, only to the extent that the research is justified by its potential prophylactic, diagnostic or therapeutic value. When medical research is combined with medical care, additional standards apply to protect the patients who are research subjects.

29. The benefits, risks, burdens and effectiveness of a new method should be tested against those of the best current prophylactic, diagnostic, and therapeutic methods. This does not exclude the use of placebo, or no treatment, in studies where no proven prophylactic, diagnostic or therapeutic method exists.

30. At the conclusion of the study, every patient entered into the study should be assured of access to the best proven prophylactic, diagnostic and therapeutic methods identified by the study.

31. The physician should fully inform the patient which aspects of the care are related to the research. The refusal of a patient to participate in a study must never interfere with the patient-physician relationship.

32. In the treatment of a patient, where proven prophylactic, diagnostic and therapeutic methods do not exist or have been ineffective, the physician, with informed consent from the patient, must be free to use unproven or new prophylactic, diagnostic and therapeutic measures, if in the physician's judgement it offers hope of saving life, re-establishing health or alleviating suffering. Where possible, these measures should be made the object of research, designed to evaluate their safety and efficacy. In all cases, new information should be recorded and, where appropriate, published. The other relevant guidelines of this Declaration should be followed.

The code outlines the principle of autonomy – the right of any person to consent voluntarily to participate in research after being fully informed [1], and to withdraw at any time from the study [9]. The research should have a clearly stated purpose, benefits should be expected [2] and the expected benefits should exceed any possible risks [6]. The research should be guided by previous knowledge [3] and be carried out by knowledgeable persons [8]. The injunction to non-malfeasance (do no harm) is contained in several clauses [4, 5, 6, 7 and 10], including the need to minimize risks when they are known [7]. The code does not specifically include an injunction to confidentiality, but this is implied in the preamble, where it is stated that experiments must "conform to the ethics of the medical profession".

All research involving human subjects should be subject to an independent ethical review carried out by institutional or national committees composed of knowledgeable persons in science, ethics and the law. Projects should be reviewed, whether they involve new drugs or procedures and whether they are physical or psychological. In all projects, the following important principles must be assured:

- Obtain informed consent for any research which involves an intervention such as a new drug or procedure [see Exercise 74].
- Ensure confidentiality of patient information [see Exercise 75].
- Enact safeguards to detect and deal with harm [see Exercise 76].
- Ensure that the study is properly designed and conducted so that a result can be expected and validated [see Exercise 77].

Special issues arise when research is being conducted in a public-health setting. There is an ethical obligation to ensure that the community will have access to any benefits that the research may bring. In certain settings, the question arises whether a community as a whole can consent through their leaders, to avoid the necessity of obtaining the consent of each individual. Many of these issues are still evolving and should be addressed through review committees of knowledgeable persons.

Exercises 74 to 77

The following scenarios are based on events in practice. Identify the ethical and legal issues and state whether the conduct of the professionals was correct and why. If the professional conduct was not correct, state what it should have been. Discussion follows the exercises.

◆ Exercise 74

Research is being conducted to determine whether the surgical excision of nail punctures is better than medical treatment for people with diabetes. The research is being conducted as a randomized trial, and the consent form requests the patient to participate in the trial of surgical excision versus medical treatment. In the protocol, the medical management proposed is Panadol.

◆ Exercise 75

Researchers have gone on national television asking for the cooperation and support of the public in carrying out a research project. They state that the study involves confidential interviews of HIV-positive subjects and their families. The interviews will be conducted by trained interviewers who will have identification cards saying they are project personnel. The protocol calls for the HIV-positive subjects to be chosen from the treatment clinic. If they consent, they will be interviewed via a questionnaire without any identifiers, and their families will also be approached for confidential interviews. The interviewers are to be paid the equivalent of US$10 for each interview and will be transported to the families' homes in the research unit's car.

◆ Exercise 76

A research group has obtained funding to do a clinical trial on a new medication. The protocol calls for the monitoring of liver function and the withdrawal of the medication should liver function deteriorate. After the study commences, the costs of the laboratory tests increase, and after discussion the research team decides to do the liver function tests only at the beginning and the end of the study.

◆ Exercise 77

A country-wide study of marijuana use among children, chosen by stratified sampling, has found that fewer than 2 per cent of children smoke marijuana. The national association STOPOT criticizes the study and calls for a study to be done by people "who know how to get information out of children". STOPOT submits a proposal for funding in which their members will interview 50 children chosen at random from among the children found on "the street that never sleeps".

Discussion

The following discussions address the issues of professional conduct raised in the exercises. Other conclusions are possible.

◆ Exercise 74

Issues

- Are the patients fully informed about the nature of the research?
- Is the study design sufficient to enable researchers to decide whether the hypothesis is true?

Professional conduct

- Patients do not appear to be informed of the nature of the medical treatment involved and therefore are not fully informed to consent to the intervention.
- The research is really designed to determine the efficacy of surgical treatment over no intervention at all, since the use of Panadol is not expected to have a therapeutic effect. The risks of providing no treatment at all must be carefully weighed and safeguards put in place to detect whether problems arise in the untreated group.

◆ Exercise 75

Issues

- Is the confidentiality of the participants sufficiently protected under the existing proposal?

Professional conduct

- There are several points at which the identity and therefore the confidentiality of the subjects with regard to their HIV status can be broken.
- The interviewers must be sworn to maintain confidentiality of the subjects' identity, not just the results of the interview.
- The driver of the vehicle will need to be sworn to maintain confidentiality of the identity of the subjects.

- Identifiers on the unit's car breach confidentiality, particularly since the researchers have identified the nature of the research project to the general public.

◆ Exercise 76

Issues

- Can the protocol of the study be changed without further approval?
- Do the changes in the protocol affect the efficacy of the study?

Professional conduct

- Before giving approval, funding agencies as well as the ethical approval committee would have considered all of the details of the study. Therefore, changes in the study should not be made without submitting them for further approval.
- The changes in the study have removed an important monitoring safeguard for the subjects involved; therefore both the ethics and the efficacy of the study have been compromised.

◆ Exercise 77

Issues

- What is the basis for the criticism of the study?
- Will the proposed study be able to answer the criticisms put forward?

Professional conduct

- It appears that the reported low prevalence of drug use is the trigger for the criticism, and the interviewers are being blamed for not being able to get the information. There appears to have been no criticism of the sampling method.
- The alternative study proposed is biased by the criticism, in that the credentials of the interviewers are not given, and it may be assumed that they share the bias of the organization. The sampling is not at all comparable and may be in fact be intended to guarantee a "better" result.

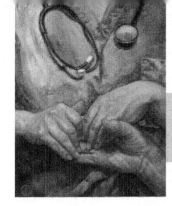

CHAPTER 10

Ethics in Public Health Practice

As members of the public become more and more aware of their health, the factors that affect it and the ethical and legal issues related to their personal health care, the ethical practices of public health practitioners also come under scrutiny. Public health is concerned with community health rather than individual illness; however, the community is made up of individuals, and their health concerns cannot be separated entirely from those of the community.

Ethical issues in public health arise where

- actions are taken to improve the health of the community as a whole, but those actions may cause harm to some individuals;
- individuals may have their liberty and autonomy denied in the interest of the public good;
- decisions have to be taken about the allocation of resources that may make some individuals or groups feel wronged;
- decisions taken to improve the public health may appear to have disadvantages in other areas of community life; or
- laws and practices intended to improve the health of the community may be disadvantageous to the individual or the community in unintended ways.

Community versus individual health risk

Public health is concerned more with prevention than with treatment, although the two cannot be divorced. Public health professionals and policy makers focus on actions in the community and monitoring of the community's health, and allocation of resources to enable both. Ethical issues arise in each of these areas of government concern, not only for the community but for the individuals within the community.

Offering vaccines to the community is intended to prevent or treat illness in the community; however, a vaccine may cause illness in an individual. If an individual health practitioner offered a vaccine without an explanation of the risks, the action would be considered unethical and negligent. Public health practitioners, in contrast, may be indemnified against adverse outcomes by the force of law, and would not necessarily think that warnings of risks were essential, either practically or ethically [see Exercise 78].

Value judgements in public health can be difficult to make outside of emergency situations, and emergency situations are probably the worst time to sort out complex value issues. Therefore, in severe public health situations, the law gives the authorities power to take action for the benefit of the community and to override individual concerns and risks. For example, public health authorities have the power to take action to control the insect vectors of serious illnesses, such as dengue or yellow fever, without regard to the effects their measures may have on an individual. If an individual in the community were to spray a poisonous substance onto another's property which affected or could affect the neighbour's health, the perpetrator could be sued for battery and endangerment of life, and a restraining order forbidding the spraying could be obtained from the court. When a public health authority does exactly the same thing to control disease-carrying insects, an individual may have no redress, even if the evidence shows that the method used does not control the insects [see Exercise 79].

Another ethical issue concerns how much responsibility health authorities should exercise in warning the community about dangers to public health. For example, if the drinking water has become unsafe, should the public be told, even if actions to correct it are contemplated? It must be considered unethical not to warn the public, particularly when the lives of vulnerable individuals, such as infants and the elderly, are in danger [see Exercise 80].

Individual liberty versus community health

Public health law may have provisions to restrict or restrain an individual against his or her will on the basis of guarding the public's health. People may be quarantined in their homes or elsewhere, restrained in designated facilities and even treated against their will. These powers place a special duty on public health authorities, and the administrators of the law that governs their actions, to safeguard the rights of the individual while safeguarding the public health.

Quarantine is the best known public health action. It has usually been imposed to deal with specific contagious diseases. Quarantine is used to minimize the risk of transmission of serious infections through casual contact or through the air, and to maintain the sick person's isolation until he or she is no longer infectious. The quarantine is lifted when the infecting organism has been eliminated from the sick person's body, either by treatment or as a result of the development of antibodies by the body's immune system. The use of quarantine may be inappropriate to deal with new diseases or different social situations from those that obtained when quarantine measures were enacted into law. For example, some people have inappropriately advocated quarantine for people infected with HIV, in spite of the fact that the disease cannot be transmitted by casual contact, there is at present no curative treatment and the body's immune response does not get rid of the virus. The result of that measure would be quarantine for life. Inappropriate measures produce an undue burden on individuals as well as the state. On the other hand, if smallpox were reintroduced, it would be entirely appropriate to quarantine affected individuals, their households and other close contacts while treatment is carried out and vaccination of the community accomplished [see Exercise 81].

There are laws passed to restrict individual liberty which are intended to safeguard individuals from themselves and reduce the risk of harm to others. Thus, although it is not against the law to drink alcohol in many jurisdictions, it is universally against the law to drive a vehicle while intoxicated, though different jurisdictions have different definitions of intoxication. Such law not only protects the individual but also reduces the risk to the community. Similarly, measures such as seat-belt and safety-helmet legislation not only reduce the extent of injury that may occur to an individual in an accident, they benefit the community by reducing the cost of treating more severe injuries, thus conserving resources. The restriction on smoking in public may not do a great deal for the individual smoker, but it does benefit the health of others who would otherwise inhale the smoke second-hand [see Exercise 82].

Allocating resources: individual versus community priorities

When authorities allocate resources to provide expensive medication or treatment to people with cancer, heart disease, HIV infection or other diseases, value judgements are often made by other ill people or their relatives about the value and priority of their own illness. For example, the relatives of a 75-year-old retired public servant who has diabetes and hypertension and is in chronic renal failure complained that authorities should not be allocating resources to the treatment of people with HIV but should use those resources to expand renal dialysis facilities, so that their relative can be treated. They justified their position on the basis that HIV is a self-inflicted disease, and HIV-positive people should not be given priority over their relative, who served the community well throughout his working life.

While individual circumstances may influence how an illness is treated, it would be ethically questionable for public policy and the allocation of resources to be based on the illness of one person. Thus, although the case of a valued former public servant may serve to make renal dialysis accessible to more people, it would be imprudent for public health officials to decide not to treat another disease on the grounds that it is self-inflicted [see Exercise 83].

Community actions with counterproductive effects

Laws that seek to protect the public, sometimes from themselves, impinge on the rights of the individual. However, there are some laws that inhibit the ability of health authorities to prevent illness. For example, criminal sanctions against intravenous drug abuse inhibit authorities from providing clean needles in exchange for used ones and thus helping prevent the spread of HIV among intravenous drug users. Similar laws inhibit the prevention and management of sexually transmitted diseases among prisoners and, to some extent, among sex workers [see Exercise 84].

Stigmatization in the community has occurred with most diseases that have a high mortality or cause an obvious disability and are difficult to treat. Stigmatization is used to discriminate against the people affected by the disease and to deny them social, economic and medical benefits that any other ill person would ordinarily expect. HIV/AIDS is the latest disease to produce major dilemmas for traditional public health practice. It demonstrates well the counterproductive role that stigmatization of a disease, and those affected by it, has on the control of disease. The stigma of HIV/AIDS has been used by some people to advocate that HIV-infected people be quarantined and denied jobs, housing and schooling. A public health rationale has also been used to deny HIV-infected persons medication on the grounds that the money it costs could be put to "better" use. Without the vigorous intervention of those affected by the stigma and some public health practitioners, a full panoply of coercive measures against HIV-affected persons would have been more widely instituted. Stigmatization deters people from finding out if they are infected, and in the case of HIV infection, affected persons who are well may unwittingly continue to spread the virus [see Exercise 85].

Advocates of the concept of "good stigma" believe that the stigmatization of smokers for the good of the community has produced a reduction in smoking. The concept is flawed, however, for smokers have not been denied legal rights, they have been separated from non-smokers only when they are smoking, and they have not been denied treatment of their addiction or its consequences, no matter how expensive. Furthermore, there is no empirical evidence to support the viewpoint that stigmatization, rather than education efforts, has reduced the prevalence of smoking.

Contraception and termination of pregnancy are considered unethical and illegal in some jurisdictions, whereas in others they are lawful measures, passed to protect the health of women in particular. Some people consider these measures responsible for the spread of sexually transmitted diseases and the development of abortion on demand, despite the inclusion in most laws of provisions to prevent such developments.

Public health authorities have a responsibility to monitor the effects of controversial public health acts and to inform the community of surveillance data so that continued actions can be supported by facts rather than uninformed opinions.

Unintended consequences

Public health actions and law should be guided by sound evidence, good epidemiological surveillance and monitoring of disease. Health authorities may sometimes be tempted to either minimize or exaggerate a situation to motivate the public. When revealed, such distortions lead to a loss of trust, and the public may stop listening or refuse to act on what may be otherwise good advice [see Exercise 86].

For example, exaggerating the negative medical effects of marijuana satisfies those who do not use it but has little, if any, effect on those who do. It probably also blunts the message about more dangerous drugs and, as a consequence, encourages rather than discourages their use. Similar consequences arise from statements that emphasize the failure rate of condoms as a contraceptive, implying an inability to protect against sexually transmitted diseases, and suggest that the only safe alternative is the widespread practice of abstinence.

Exercises 78 to 86

The following scenarios are based on events in practice. Identify the ethical and legal issues and state whether the conduct of the professionals was correct and why. If the professional conduct was not correct, state what it should have been. Discussion follows the exercises.

◈ Exercise 78

The ministry of health has announced a mass campaign to combat an epidemic in the country through administration of an oral vaccine containing a live attenuated virus. The medical association has warned the public about taking the vaccine, on the grounds that in another country it produced the disease itself in 1 of every 750,000 people who got the vaccine. The medical association says that the injectable killed vaccine is safe and should be used instead. The ministry responds that the oral vaccine was chosen because it could be administered quickly and at little cost, and that the risk associated with the oral vaccine is negligible.

◈ Exercise 79

The government has passed a law intended to promote recycling of waste and cleaning up of the environment. One of the provisions is that no one may buy a new car battery unless the old one is returned. The law also mandates that items containing lead and mercury must not be disposed of at the solid-waste dump, along the roadside or in the sea. During the debate in parliament, the government has stated that batteries that cannot be recycled by the local company should be brought to be burned at the public incinerator. After the measure has passed, Dr Read writes to the press, stating that the policy will cause damage to the health of children through the inhalation of lead-containing smoke and calling for the repeal of the entire law as misdirected and a danger to public health.

◈ Exercise 80

Mrs Onway lives in a house that is badly in need of repair. Her neighbours have complained to the ministry of health that the house is rat-infested and that the rats come onto their property, and they are worried that the rats might carry disease. The public health inspectors visit Mrs Onway and tell her she must clean up the property and put down rat bait. Mrs Onway replies, "You think I going pay Miss Nosy any mind? Tell she if she has rats that they coming from right under she bed."

Exercise 81

Dr Risk was not feeling well when he got up in the morning, and when he was having his shower he noticed a pustule on his left side. He mentions it to his wife, who works in the paediatric department of the hospital, and she remarks, "That's exactly how chickenpox starts; we had a number of cases recently. You never did get the vaccine when I asked you to do it a month ago." She advises him to stay home, but he responds that the department is short of staff and he will take some Panadol, go and do the ward round, get some acyclovir from the pharmacy and come back home as soon as the ward round is finished.

Exercise 82

In between operations, Dr Cutright goes into a nearby office and lights up a cigarette. Dr Blowharde comes into the office and says to the secretary, "Someone move the No Smoking sign from off the door?" The secretary says, "No," and Dr Cutright remarks, "There is no law in this country against smoking, so you might as well take down the sign."

Exercise 83

The government has announced the acquisition of a laser at the cost of $250,000 and says this will bring the country into line with modern surgical care, allowing surgery to be done with less scarring and pain. Dr Foote, in an interview after the announcement, welcomes the purchase of the equipment but wonders why government continues to ignore a repeated request for equipment, costing half as much, to measure the blood supply in the feet of people with diabetes, which would help to prevent the large number of amputations in the country.

Exercise 84

Seat-belt legislation has been passed by the government, and Dr Nohall writes a letter to the press, stating, "Admirable as the government may feel in that it is saving us from ourselves, what the public has not been told about is the danger of seat belts. Some years ago you would have seen a newspaper report where a car overturned and the driver was trapped behind the wheel and as a result was burnt to a cinder. Furthermore, doctors at the hospital have seen a number of cases of ruptured intestines as this 'life-saver' tightens you in its grip. The CMO should have the courage to speak out and not hide under the skirts of the minister."

◆ Exercise 85

There has been a series of articles in the press about obesity and its adverse effects. The minister of health has said in an address that his ministry is preparing a cabinet paper calling for banning the importation of all white flour and products made from it. He states that we have been following the bad eating habits of the white people for too long and we need to get back to the traditional foods. The policy will encourage farmers to grow a greater variety of crops and it will demonstrate government's commitment to an integrated food and health policy. When asked to comment, the Chamber of Commerce says that the policy will force a lot of businesses like bakeries and fast-food restaurants to close down.

◆ Exercise 86

Dr Whytehorn writes to the press to say that, based on his survey of the sexual practices of black patients in the public clinic, half of the population will have AIDS in five years' time. He says everyone should stop having sex and get tested, and those who test positive should be tattooed and carry a photo ID card. The advisory committee to the government takes issue with the doctor's conclusions and warns that such alarmist tactics will do more harm than good.

Discussion

The following discussions address the issues of professional conduct raised in the exercises. Other conclusions are possible.

◆ Exercise 78

Issues

- Is it ethical for the government to use a measure that has a small but definite risk when a safer alternative is available?
- Should the medical association intervene on such matters and advise the public to not cooperate with the public health authorities?

Professional conduct

- Members of the community should be given enough information to enable them to consent to any medical measure that is being offered, whether by a surgeon or a public health practitioner. Public health authorities should therefore reveal any risks that are associated with a measure they advocate and balance them against the risks of not taking the measure.

- When costs are a determining factor in a decision, these should also be explained and an attempt made to explain the cost effectiveness to the public.
- The medical association has a duty to comment on matters that affect their members, and illness in the community is therefore a matter of concern. However, they should calculate the risk-benefit ratio of their advice. For example, if one person were to become ill with the vaccine offered by the government, but half the population elected not to be vaccinated and 50 people were affected by the disease, the advice would have done more harm than good.

Exercise 79

Issues

- Are intrusive regulations necessary to protect the public from lead and mercury poisoning?
- Is it correct that incineration of batteries will endanger the health of children?
- What are the alternatives for safe disposal?

Professional conduct

- The determination to protect the public health from lead and mercury poisoning should be based on a scientific study of the extent of the current problem and the best means by which to protect the public. Any regulations should then be based on scientific advice and not on arguments made during parliamentary debate.
- If Dr Read is correct that incineration is not safe, then the regulation is faulty and should be revisited and changed depending on the scientific advice. It should not be necessary to scrap the entire legislation if only one provision is at fault.
- When regulations are being considered, consultation should first be held with all relevant persons – the public, representatives from the specific industry involved and members of the scientific and professional community.

Exercise 80

Issues

- Should the public health authorities have responded to the complaint in the way they did?
- Should the public health authorities reveal the origin of a complaint?
- Do the authorities have the power to compel a person to follow their advice?

Professional conduct

- The public health authorities have a duty to respond to any threat to public health, no matter how the threat comes to their attention. Rats do carry a risk to public health. However, the authorities should assess the nature of the threat rather than simply take a complainant's word for it.

- Threats to public health should be anticipated and a surveillance system put in place. An efficient system of checking derelict properties that might be a breeding place for rats should obviate the need for the kind of personal complaint illustrated in the case.

- Public health authorities should not identify complainants who bring a situation to their attention. The complainant's identity should be kept confidential, for it could give rise to interpersonal conflict. In the case described, such a breach might not have occurred, for there apparently had been previous exchanges between the two neighbours.

- The "threat" should be thoroughly investigated and the evidence for the conclusion made available to the householder. In this case, what is the evidence for the rats being present and their origin? Have the authorities looked at the complainant's premises with the same "eyes"?

- Public health law usually has provisions to compel citizens/householders to comply with their advice. This may extend, after due notice, to demolishing derelict premises or to requiring offenders to pay for such actions as clearing bush from their premises.

◆ Exercise 81

Issues

- Should doctors self-diagnose and decide on what actions to take?
- Is the doctor knowingly putting others at risk?
- Should all doctors be vaccinated against known risks?
- Is a doctor liable if a patient gets a disease from the doctor during the course of treatment?
- What responsibility, if any, does the wife have in this matter?
- What if this were an emergency situation?

Professional conduct

- Self-diagnosis is fraught with problems: objectivity is usually lacking, and judgements may be made that are convenient to the doctor. In the case of transmissible disease, it is particularly inappropriate, for, as in this case, the doctor may make a decision that could result in transmission to patients and colleagues.

The decision to go to work on the putative self-diagnosis is flawed in two ways, for if the doctor decided not to go to work, in the absence of independent confirmation of the diagnosis he could be accused of shirking.

- Doctors should not put others at risk for transmissible diseases, particularly as they may be dealing with very ill patients whose lives may be endangered by another infection. In the case described, colleagues are also being put at risk, and this may make the shortage of staff even worse. Doctors should be aware that some diseases may have severe sequelae in otherwise well persons, such as their colleagues.

- Public health authorities should insist that all health workers be vaccinated against all transmissible diseases, as protection for both the worker and the patients for whom he or she is responsible.

- Knowingly putting others at risk can certainly lead to a suit of negligence, no matter how well-intentioned the doctor may have been. When one is ill, judgement may be impaired, and this is another reason for seeking independent advice.

- The wife is evidently knowledgeable in the field but has not insisted that her husband stay at home. This illustrates that, as with self-diagnosis, advice within the close family circle may not be completely objective. A sick doctor may put the diagnosis and the risks to others in the recesses of his or her mind and may even formulate an alternative diagnosis to allow the intended actions to be pursued. The wife, as a doctor herself, should have insisted on her husband's staying at home or getting independent advice; she also should have considered what action to take regarding her own possibly infected status.

- One can justify a risk of transmitting disease only in an emergency where there is no other professional who could undertake the intended tasks. Such a situation is highly unlikely except in the most remote locations, and even then, the alternative of evacuating the patient must be considered.

◆ Exercise 82

Issues

- Should smoking be allowed in a health-care institution?
- Is a law required to ban smoking in a private or public place?
- Should professional colleagues react in the manner described?

Professional conduct

- It is difficult to justify smoking by anyone in a health-care institution, particularly in the presence of patients or in a situation such as the case described, where there appears to have been a determination that it should not take place.

- Whether or not there is a law that bans smoking in the country, institutions and businesses can formulate enforceable rules within the institution. Assuming that the No Smoking sign was not put on the door arbitrarily by an individual but rather by the person responsible for the department, it should be respected as if it had the force of law. Some organizations set aside specially designated areas for those who smoke.
- The interaction between the professionals appears inappropriate, in the sense that they do not address the problem face to face but through a third party who is in a subordinate position. This form of indirect interaction probably reflects an unresolved conflict between the two professionals, and their way of dealing with it will probably not resolve the issue.

◆ *Exercise 83*

Issues

- How are resources allocated?
- Should allocation of resources be examined in public?
- How do donations factor into resource allocation?

Professional conduct

- Resources are usually allocated through an administrative mechanism that considers a number of factors, including individual influence, departmental requests and administrative or political priorities. There should be a discernible rationale, based on need and the financial resources available. In the case cited, the anticipated benefits of the laser appear to affect a broad cross-section of patients, but the problems they will address – pain and scarring associated with surgery – do not appear to be as critical as the problem of too many amputations.
- There should be room for an expression of divergent views. However, in some systems there are rules intended to prohibit such public expressions. Advocacy on behalf of patients is a good thing, although it should not be done in such a way as to suggest that patients are competing. In this case, the statement welcomes the equipment but clearly suggests that there are more important priorities.
- Donations for specific purposes may clash with established priorities. When this happens, the conflict should be discussed candidly with the proposed donor to try to resolve the concerns. In accepting donations, institutions should make the wishes of the donor clearly known, in case a suggestion arises that the authorities have misplaced priorities.

Exercise 84

Issues

- Are the doctor's claims true, and, if so, should the legislation be enforced?
- How should the authorities handle this criticism?

Professional conduct

- There are advantages and disadvantages to every action. The doctor has written to stress the disadvantages of wearing seat belts but has not said whether there are any advantages. Legislative action should be based on studies of the problem and the outcomes, where available, of the measures proposed, not on a one-sided analysis of the issue.
- Outcome measures must indicate that the outcome of taking the proposed action is significantly better than that of not doing so, and outcomes must be monitored to ensure that the expected advantages are realized and that the significance of any disadvantages that do arise is measured.
- The authorities should have had available the studies on which the legislation is based and relevant local figures on the issue. These should be published so that the public understands both sides of the issue.

Exercise 85

Issues

- Are the policy objectives worthy?
- Will the proposed policy achieve its objectives?
- Are the cultural changes envisaged in the policy desirable and achievable?
- Are the objections valid?

Professional conduct

- Reducing obesity sounds like a worthy objective, but it is not clear that all of the factors contributing to obesity have been taken into account. The ministry appears to be taking into account only the caloric contribution of a single food item.
- The proposed policy does not appear to be viable as stated, given the fact that it covers only one aspect of the reasons for obesity. Little attention seems to have been given to what alternative to white flour will be recommended, and whether the alternative will contribute to the reduction in obesity.
- The notion that such a simplistic solution can bring about a cultural change is naïve. There is also a call on racial issues as a motivator for change. If the intention

is to bring about an association in people's minds between white flour and "white" culture, the use of the phrase can be seen as race baiting.

- The objections from the Chamber of Commerce seem alarmist and as simplistic as the proposed policy, for there is nothing adduced to say that alternatives will not be found, particularly other forms of flour.

◆ Exercise 86

Issues

- Does the doctor have the right to write to the public about findings in the public clinic?
- Can the doctor draw those conclusions from what he has studied?
- Is the doctor trying to induce fear in the community to get his advice followed?
- Does fear work as a motivator?
- Are the measures proposed practical or ethical?
- Is the response of the advisory committee appropriate?

Professional conduct

- The public service usually has rules prohibiting doctors from speaking about problems in the service without permission. Where such rules exist, they should not be used to inhibit genuine research findings that are of public interest. The racial content in the remarks may be either a straightforward description of the clinic population or a conscious effort to highlight a difference in sexual behaviour between the races. The characterization of black people as sexually promiscuous is a well-known racist stereotype, and this may have to be considered when assessing the validity of the study.
- Insufficient detail is given to substantiate the conclusions drawn. With such stark conclusions, it is incumbent on the doctor to give enough details of the study methods so that its validity can be assessed.
- From the remarks reported, there can be no conclusion drawn other than that the doctor wishes to induce fear.
- Except as a motivator for flight from danger, fear has not been shown to motivate appropriate behavioural change. This is best illustrated by a fire, when an orderly exit is required but is often replaced by stampeding. If there is research that shows that fear motivates changes in sexual behaviour, the doctor should have offered it with the remarks.
- The proposed measures appear expensive and impractical, and are reminiscent of measures used historically by repressive regimes against people of specific classes, races or faiths. It is unethical to discriminate against people with illness in the community. If illness justifies separation from the community, it must be carried

out within the law by public health authorities. Isolation, or quarantine, is usually imposed only to prevent transmission of contagious diseases.

- The advisory committee's response is appropriate, given the facts and studies used to counter the doctor's contentions. Time will tell who is right, but sometimes one should not wait, if there are other studies elsewhere that can be used to draw conclusions.

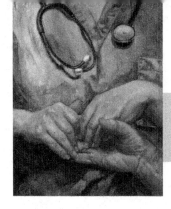

Case Studies

When ethical or legal problems arise in health care, they are seldom isolated problems, for the incorrect handling of a situation frequently produces other problems. Incorrect conduct is usually discovered by the problem it produces, and health-care workers may compound the problem by taking inappropriate actions in an attempt to cover over the original problem.

The following case studies are based on problems that have arisen in practice. They have been altered to remove any identification of patients or professionals involved. However, the essence of the cases is preserved to illustrate the reality of how the problems emerged.

Each case report is followed by identification and discussion of the issues involved. The opinions given in the case analyses are those of the author and have been discussed either at an ethical committee or a case conference.

Refusal to consent

Case report

A 69-year-old woman was admitted to hospital with a gangrenous foot. She lived alone, and during a visit her niece had noticed an offensive smell coming from her foot and, over the aunt's protestations, had called the ambulance. The patient was unkempt and uncooperative but was quiet, refusing to talk at times. She was not known to have diabetes or hypertension.

On examination she was not ill-looking but was febrile. There was wet gangrene of the left forefoot, with pulses felt in both limbs except in the affected foot. She was placed on antibiotics, the foot was dressed and she was advised to have it amputated, which she refused.

The day after admission the relatives advised that the patient had a history of mental disease and had been institutionalized 15 years before. The patient continued to refuse surgery and was referred for a psychiatric consultation. On the second day after admission she was seen by the consultant psychiatrist, who noted paranoid ideation with some insight into her current medical illness. The patient was reported to say, among other things, "I don't trust anyone."

By the eighth day after admission, the offensive smell persisted but there were no other signs of sepsis, and the gangrene had not extended further. In spite of the urging of relatives and staff, the patient continued to refuse amputation. On review, the psychiatrist concluded that the patient's psychosis prevented her from making rational decisions.

Another surgeon was asked to see the patient, agreed with the need for amputation and suggested that the foot be exposed so that the patient could see the situation for herself.

Five weeks after admission, the psychiatrist suggested commencement of anti-psychotic medication, with a view to monitoring clinical progress and also with the hope that the patient would gain insight into the nature of her foot problem. After six days of medication, she remained grossly thought-disordered, was less objectionable and more approachable, but remained adamant that she wanted no surgery.

At eight weeks after admission, the forefoot had mummified with a line of demarcation. She complained of mild foot pain and still insisted that the surgeons wanted to hurt her, not help her. The psychiatrist concluded that she was mentally unfit to take care of herself and recommended that proceedings be commenced for her involuntary admission to the psychiatric hospital.

Ethical and legal issues

"The medical judgement that treatment is indicated does not entail the ethical judgement that it ought to be administered to a particular patient. Judgements of medical indication do not command the patient or doctor categorically but give medical advice" (Miller 1993).

The law regarding refusal of treatment

A legally and mentally competent patient has an absolute right to consent to anything that is done to him or her. This includes matters that may be considered non-threatening or trivial to health-care staff, as well as matters that may threaten the patient's life. Refusal of treatment or investigation by a competent patient can be overridden only by an order in court. The remedies available to the patient who is treated against his or her will are a charge of battery or a suit of negligence.

In the case described, the patient refused the proffered surgical treatment but accepted all other treatment measures. The information about her psychotic illness, offered by the relatives after she has refused surgery, clearly raises the question of her ability to give informed consent to, or refuse, treatment. Clear documentation of the patient's refusal, the explanations given for the advice and the efforts made to persuade the patient should be placed in the notes.

Informed consent

To be valid in law, consent must be informed, meaning that the patient should know and understand what is to happen. This means that the diagnosis, general nature of the proposed procedure, anticipated benefits and risks, and alternatives should be explained. Explanations have to be in terms that the patient can understand. In the case described, the question was clearly raised of whether the patient was able to understand her condition and the treatment being offered. However, apart from surgery she appeared to accept all other treatment and was cooperative in every other respect.

The consultant psychiatrist who saw her first concluded that she had "paranoid ideation" but also stated that she had some insight into her illness. No medication was initially ordered for the psychiatric disorder, which would lead one to conclude that it was not thought that she would improve with medication and that she was not considered a threat to herself or others. One may well ask what was expected from the psychiatric consultation – that the psychiatrist could persuade the patient to accept the operation, or that the psychiatrist's opinion could overrule that of the patient if the patient was deemed mentally incompetent?

The law and mental incompetence

If an adult patient is unable to consent – for example, if the person is in a coma – the next of kin or the person in charge of an institution responsible for the patient may consent. The mental capacity of a patient can change from time to time, and a patient may be able to understand simple situations but not those that are more complex.

Family members are not legally entitled to speak on an adult patient's behalf unless they have been appointed the patient's legal guardian. The legal guardian of a mentally incapacitated patient has the power to consent to treatment for the patient. In matters such as consenting to the treatment of illness, it is usually accepted that the next of kin may consent for the incapacitated patient; however, when dealing with situations where property is involved, it is wise to ensure that the relative is the legal guardian.

Incompetence as a result of mental illness is usually determined by the provisions of specific legislation in the relevant jurisdiction. For example, under the provisions of the Mental Health Act (1980) in Barbados, a person who is involuntarily admitted to the psychiatric hospital (or other place authorized by the minister of health) can be deemed by the medical superintendent to be incapable of giving informed consent, and psychiatric treatment can be administered without consent. Similar provisions exist in most jurisdictions.

Mentally incapacitated patients are entitled to treatment of conditions other than psychiatric illness when such treatment is in their best interest. If necessary, the best interest of the patient may have to be established in court. If there is a difference of opinion, it is best to discuss the matter with all parties and to come to an agreement without invoking the law.

In the case under consideration, had the patient been delirious from sepsis, the relatives would have been asked to sign the consent form, for it is easier to determine mental incapacity to consent when it is caused by common conditions such as sepsis or hypoxia than to determine incapacity from mental illness. In this case, two psychiatrists differed on whether the patient's psychosis required treatment, and after three weeks of medication "involuntary admission documentation was initiated".

The law in emergencies

Any doctor may act in the best interest of a patient in an emergency situation where the patient's life is threatened. The "best interest" cannot be for the benefit of someone else – such as putting the patient on a ventilator in the hope of the patient becoming an organ donor, or not using a ventilator because it is anticipated that someone more "worthy" may require it.

In the case described, the doctors' judgement initially was that an amputation was needed urgently, but the patient's condition was not an immediate threat to life. The patient was not incapacitated by delirium from her sepsis, and although she expressed paranoid feelings, particularly about the doctors, she appeared sufficiently lucid to convince all concerned that she understood what an amputation was and that she did not want it performed.

What course of action should have been taken if she had become septicaemic and her life was then in immediate danger? If the patient, upon admission, had been septicaemic, delirious and in danger of her life, the relatives would have been asked to give consent. In the case under consideration, however, the patient firmly objected to the operation, and her clearly expressed wishes, given that she was aware of the possible consequences, should prevail.

Prior wishes

Given the patient's right to autonomy over his or her body, the patient's wishes, clearly expressed, should be respected. This is usually invoked in regard to whether a patient should be resuscitated or placed on ventilation, should certain situations arise. This is the purpose for which advanced directives such as living wills have been used. Living wills, like DNR orders, are sometimes not respected, because health-care workers faced with emergency situations often feel compelled to safeguard themselves legally during the crisis and argue about the patient's wishes later.

In the case described, the patient clearly expressed her wishes, but there was a question about her ability to make a rational decision. In such a case, the only safe course would be to let a court decide. Medical situations, however, can become urgent quickly, and there may not be enough time to argue effectively before the court. If the patient's next of kin and relatives definitely want the doctors to proceed in spite of the patient's wishes, the legal ground might be firmer but will not prevent a legal challenge by the patient on recovery. This raises the question of whether the doctors, by consenting to the patient's wishes, are a party to a suicidal act by the patient.

To "commit suicide" by refusing treatment

Suicide is an illegal act, and doctors, apart from saving lives, should prevent and not be a party to illegal acts, wherever possible. However, suicide is an act of commission; it is not normally considered to be an act of omission. Humans are mortal and all of us will die from an illness of some sort; few will argue that people should not have some say about the manner in which they will die.

There is a community interest in preventing unnecessary deaths, and an equally strong individual interest in the quality of one's life. Therefore, each case would have to be argued on its merits. For example, a court in the United States ordered that a woman, a Jehovah's Witness with dependent children, should have a blood transfusion against her wishes, in order that she might live for the benefit of her children. A similar case was decided in the opposite manner because it was pointed out that the children would be well looked after by relatives (Meisel 1992). Normally a court will allow a competent adult to refuse treatment even if it will result in death.

In the case described, the situation did not arise – in fact, the patient confounded medical opinion and improved rather than getting worse. It would be difficult to speculate on what arguments could be put before a court to support the position that this patient's wishes should not be respected, for her mental illness was not initially judged as impairing her decision-making ability, or what would be the "community's interest" in her having an amputation.

The patient's best interest

The best interest of a patient must take into account both mental and physical status and the effect that any actual or anticipated disability will have on the quality of life. It appears from the description of this patient's living conditions that a major amputation would make her situation worse. Nevertheless, living conditions could be improved and services provided to give an amputee an acceptable quality of life. It could be concluded that, if they are to override this particular patient's wishes, the relatives or the community should be obliged to improve the conditions under which she lives and to ensure treatment for her mental condition.

Changing the patient's mind

What measures can be used to persuade a patient to change his or her mind? Counselling by health-care workers and priests, discussion with relatives and friends, and obtaining a second opinion are all fair and acceptable methods. However, counselling has risks if done inexpertly and if the patient's best interest is not the primary focus. Coercive measures, such as withholding medication or other items of care or threatening to discharge the patient, are not ethically acceptable.

Because the outcome of medical treatment is not absolute, some measures that are coercive in one circumstance may be within the normal standard of practice in other situations; it is the intention behind the advice that becomes an ethical issue.

In the case under consideration, second opinions, both psychiatric and surgical, were sought, and the patient was urged by both relatives and nursing staff to accept medical advice. The second psychiatric opinion advised medication with the intent of altering the patient's mental state to see if she would then comply with advice. Such an intention could be hazardous both ethically and legally, particularly if the patient is sedated when she makes a decision or if the patient's wishes are overridden while she is incapacitated by sedation. In the event, the medication had the effect of making the patient more approachable but did not change her mind.

The second surgical opinion reaffirmed the surgical advice and advised that as a "persuasive" measure, the gangrenous limb should be exposed so that the patient could see how futile refusal was. In some instances, it is acceptable and standard treatment to expose a gangrenous part while awaiting demarcation of the dead part from the rest of the body. The issue that arises here is that this was not the intent of the exposure. In the event, exposure did not alter the patient's mind but probably offended both staff and patients in the ward. This raises the question of whether treatment can be mandated for the "protection" of others.

For the benefit of others

Can refusal of treatment be overridden if there is a threat to others? There are provisions in both public health regulations and mental health acts to protect the public from a patient who is a risk to the public and refuses treatment for the relevant disorder. The authorized medical officer would have the power under public health regulations to confine or isolate patients for prescribed communicable disorders and to enter premises or destroy property that is deemed to be a public health hazard. Mental health acts and the courts provide for the restraint and treatment of a mentally ill person who is a deadly threat to a third party, the community or themselves.

In the case described, there was no notifiable communicable disease treatable by amputation; neither was there any question of the patient being a threat to others physically, in spite of her mental condition. The complaint of an offensive odour amounts to one of public nuisance. A public nuisance such as an offensive odour does impinge on the rights of patients, staff and visitors to the ward. To coerce an amputation on such grounds, however, is both ethically and legally indefensible when there are other ways in which the public nuisance could be removed. For example, measures could be used to limit the growth of the odour-causing bacteria, or the patient could be moved to a less "public" environment. The medical measures accepted by the patient did eventually reduce the infection and the consequential public nuisance.

Patients should be persuaded rather than coerced into accepting medical advice.

> The physician knows the many clinical distinctions that tell him when death is imminent or hope abundant; when to treat and when to wait; when to sedate with drugs and when to sedate with words; when to stop treatment, change or add; when to treat aggressively for cure, palliatively for relief and consolingly for comfort. . . . But he cannot express these specifically or consistently. (Feinstein 1994)

HIV pregnancy and a premature infant

Case report

Ms Lott was brought to the accident and emergency department with a seizure. She was 18 years old and 26 weeks pregnant. She was HIV-positive, her blood group was B positive and her venereal disease research laboratory slide test (VDRL) was non-reactive. She was on a Nevaripine protocol to reduce the risk of perinatal transmission of HIV. This was her second pregnancy; the first one had occurred while she was still at school and had been terminated.

This pregnancy had been uneventful until she had the seizure. She was initially assessed as having eclampsia with possible intrauterine foetal death. An ultrasound showed a single intrauterine pregnancy with a breech presentation; no foetal movement was seen, and there was sluggish cardiac activity. Her blood pressure ranged from 144 to 156 systolic over 82 to 93 diastolic. She was started on hydralazine and magnesium sulfate to lower her blood pressure, and induction of labour was attempted and failed four times. A caesarean section was arranged.

On being given the reasons for doing a caesarean section, she stated that if her baby did not survive she would attempt to have another. When delivered, the baby was pale and floppy, there was no spontaneous respiration and the heart rate was less than 100 beats per minute. Manual ventilation by bagging was commenced, but there was no improvement in the heart rate within 30 seconds. The baby was intubated, and positive pressure ventilation and cardiac compressions were commenced. Improvement in the baby's colour was noted after 5 minutes, and full resuscitation efforts were continued. By 19 minutes of life, the baby had developed spontaneous respiration. The endotracheal tube was removed, and the baby was given free-flow oxygen. The APGAR scores were 1(1) 1(3) 1(5) 6(19), and by 23 minutes there was minimal activity.

The infant was transferred to the neonatal intensive care unit. Findings on examination were birth weight of 900 grams, pink mucous membranes, delayed capillary refill, tachypnoea, decreased breath sounds bilaterally, and floppy tone but otherwise normal; gestation was assessed at 29 weeks. The infant was treated intensively for hyaline membrane disease and sepsis, receiving two blood transfusions and multiple antibiotics. During the baby's stay on the ward, the father visited regularly, showed great care and concern for the baby and, on one occasion, was found looking in the notes. The infant, weighing 1,590 grams, was discharged on day 59 on Vidaylin, Galfer and Eprex.

Ethical and legal issues

Age at first pregnancy

The patient is on her second pregnancy at the age of 18 years, which in the jurisdiction is the age of majority. The age of consent to sexual intercourse in the jurisdiction is 16 years, and compulsory schooling finishes at that age. Since she was still at school when her first pregnancy was terminated, it is likely that she was under the age of 16 years; intercourse between an adult and a child under 16 could be prosecuted under the provisions of the law against statutory rape.

Although a girl can consent to intercourse at the age of 16 and presumably is capable of becoming pregnant, between the ages of 16 and 18 years the parents or guardians are still legally responsible for making medical decisions on her behalf. However, under the provisions of the law in some jurisdictions – for example, the Medical Termination of Pregnancy Act (1983) in Barbados – a 16-year-old can take the decision to terminate a pregnancy of up to 12 weeks' gestation without parental permission. In addition, a child who has been pregnant may be treated as a liberated minor and can be given contraceptives without her parents' knowledge or consent if the child requests confidentiality and the doctor feels that respecting her confidentiality is in the child's best interest [*Gillick v. West Norfolk Area Health Authority* 3 A.E.R. 402 (1985)].

Termination of pregnancy in a minor

In jurisdictions where termination of pregnancy is legal, the law usually calls for the patient to be counselled. At the time of counselling, advice should be given about contraception and also about HIV. Counselling should not be seen as simply satisfying the terms of the law but should be followed with additional counselling to prevent further problems, including HIV infection.

If, as it appears in this case, the first pregnancy occurred when the patient was still a minor, the termination of her pregnancy should not have been done without the consent of her parents or guardian, unless the doctor was relying on the Gillick precedent and decided that it was in the child's best interest for the parents not to know. In any case, the doctor looking after the child should have initiated HIV counselling and tried to obtain permission for HIV testing.

Antenatal HIV testing

Jurisdictions vary as to whether HIV testing of pregnant women is mandatory or voluntary. In most jurisdictions it is voluntary, out of concern that mandatory testing may lead to a delay in the pregnant woman's seeking antenatal care. Where antiretroviral treatment is available and affordable, voluntary testing is very effective, and, with good counselling, ensures the cooperation of HIV-positive women with all of the complex measures that are necessary to combat the spread of the disease. HIV testing should be preceded by pre-test counselling; if the test turns out to be positive, the woman should have post-test counselling as well.

If the patient under discussion had received HIV testing and counselling at the time of the termination of her first pregnancy, she should have been educated not only about HIV but about the risk of transmission of the disease through the unprotected intercourse required to become pregnant again, as well as the problems associated with an HIV-positive infant. The fact that a young girl comes to her second pregnancy HIV-positive indicates that the education and counselling that should have been done at the time of her first pregnancy was ineffective and should be reviewed.

Counselling

Counselling offered in conjunction with pregnancy termination or HIV testing is intended to educate women about the risks of these conditions, and to advise and persuade them to use contraception and to practise safer sex for the primary and secondary prevention of HIV. In the case of HIV-positive women, counselling should seek to empower them to avoid spreading HIV to others and to inform, or accept assistance in informing, their sexual contacts.

In the case of a pregnant woman, there is both a present and a future risk of transmission of HIV to the infant and to the sexual partners with whom she has unprotected sex. The situation is further complicated in those places where the government medical service offers antiretroviral treatment only to pregnant women and only for a period during the pregnancy, with the sole intention of reducing the rate of transmission from mother to child.

Counselling also has to prepare people with HIV to deal with the stigma and discrimination that are the lot of the HIV-positive person, and with the lethal consequences of AIDS should they be unable to afford treatment. Counselling should therefore be done by a trained person if it is to be effective in achieving its aims, whether they are to encourage HIV testing and contraceptive use or to help HIV-positive people deal with the realities of the disease. Failure to achieve the aims of counselling should signal that either the method or the resources are not working as intended and should be reviewed.

Some may feel that the determination of the patient in the case report to have another child, knowing that she is HIV-positive, represents a failure of the counselling effort. This judgement cannot be made without a knowledge of all of the facts, including the HIV status of her sexual partner and the extended family's ability and willingness to look after a child should the parents die. Furthermore, the innate desire to reproduce should not be underestimated, and in such cases professionals may have to turn their attention to how reproduction can be achieved safely and in the long-term interest of all the parties involved.

The father

A commonly heard witticism is "Maternity is a fact, paternity is an act of faith." Who is the father? The father is the person whom the mother identifies as the father and who acknowledges it. Legally, he is the spouse, the adoptive parent or the person who registers his name on the birth certificate. In cases of dispute regarding the identity of the biological father, DNA testing can be done.

Identification of the father in the first pregnancy in this case is important, because if the girl was less than 16 years old and the father was an adult, he would be liable for a charge of statutory rape. However, in many jurisdictions the charge of statutory rape is seldom pursued since the child is unwilling to give evidence. In some instances, the girl's parents may be unwilling to pursue a case because the father – the "sugar daddy" – is providing financial support for the home.

The father may also be the person who passed on HIV infection to the girl. It is therefore important to seek to diagnose the HIV status of the father and to provide the necessary education and counselling to prevent the further spread of the virus. If it is discovered that the person knew that he was HIV-positive, consideration should be given to prosecution.

In some jurisdictions there are specific laws dealing with the wilful transmission of HIV. However, most countries have other laws that deal with causing harm to others, ranging from causing bodily harm to murder, and people have been prosecuted under them. A typical act used is an Offences Against the Person Act. The one in Barbados (1995) states: "Any person who unlawfully and maliciously or recklessly engages in conduct which places, or may place, another person in danger of death or serious bodily harm is guilty of an offence and is liable on conviction on indictment to imprisonment for life."

The rights of the father

Does the father have the right to know the mother's HIV status? The mother has the right to confidentiality; however, through supportive counselling she must be encouraged to inform her sexual partner(s) of her status. This would also involve expert counselling of the partner before he (or they) is subjected to testing. Such counselling would also need to stress the male's responsibility to any other sexual partners he may have.

If the mother's HIV-positive status was detected before this pregnancy and she did not let her sexual partner know, then there is good legal precedent to breach her confidentiality and let the partner know without her consent. However, one must always be conscious of the complexities innate in any relationship, and particularly issues of economic support, in making decisions on these delicate matters.

Do the health-care staff have a role in protecting the father's health? Staff have an obligation to look at the HIV status of all the sexual contacts of an HIV-positive person, and this is best done with confidentiality and the cooperation of the HIV-positive person. The staff have the right to warn any sexual contacts who have been knowingly put at risk. It is therefore vital to know when the HIV status was known and if the risk behaviour continued after that time.

In the case under discussion, there are opportunities for counselling and testing the father: it is likely that a blood transfusion will be required, and the subject of HIV testing could be introduced in the context of the father's being a possible blood donor. However, blood should not be accepted from the father, even if he tests HIV-negative, unless he has not had sexual intercourse with the mother in the last three months. In spite of improvement in the sensitivity of HIV tests, there is still a "window" period for seroconversion. With the current state of testing, three months should be a safe period, although most people who become infected will seroconvert within six weeks.

What right does the father have to information about the baby? The father has the legal right to all information about his child. Therefore, when a baby is born HIV-positive the father should be told, irrespective of the indirect breach of the confidentiality of the mother's status. This is a situation that requires a choice between competing rights, and the father's rights could be said to outweigh those of the mother since she should have informed him about her status.

HIV and pregnancy

Women have the right to autonomy and to consent to sexual intercourse – and, presumably, thereby to reproduce – once they reach the legal age of consent. However, reproduction involves responsibilities of the father and responsibilities of both parents to the baby, and these must be taken into account when conflict arises.

The autonomy of persons can be proscribed in law, but there is nothing in the law denying a woman the right to reproduce, and there is a strong desire to pass on one's genes, particularly when one feels under threat. Nonetheless, an HIV-positive woman needs to be counselled with respect to all of the problems the child will face, and the risk to which she exposes her sexual partner if he is not also HIV-positive. An HIV-positive woman expressing the desire for a child should be encouraged to reveal her HIV status to her partner, and if she does not, there is a strong case for breaching her confidentiality and warning the third party if that party is known. There may be more than one partner, and it is possible for the woman to simply change partners if she strongly desires to have a child. There is an alternative to risking transmission to an HIV-negative sexual partner: artificial insemination.

Should treatment be different when a complication arises? Pregnant women should be treated with the same standard of care regardless of their HIV status. Not all infants born to HIV-positive mothers will be infected with HIV, and those who are not should have the opportunities of any other child who is not HIV-positive. The use of antiretroviral therapy in the perinatal period has reduced the rate of transmission of HIV from the mother to the infant from between 15 and 40 per cent to between 3 and 10 per cent. In the absence of antiretroviral therapy, a caesarean section is said to reduce the risk of HIV infection during the birth process.

It is surprising that the pre-eclamptic state of the patient under discussion was not recognized when she presented with a seizure. One might also ask whether, with a live but distressed infant, it is normal practice to make several attempts to induce labour.

Should an HIV-positive woman be offered caesarean section? The use of a C-section to reduce the risk of transmission in the absence of perinatal antiretroviral therapy is often a moot point, for in those countries that cannot afford perinatal therapy, an increase in the number of elective caesarean sections usually cannot be afforded either. Therefore, the decision to do a C-section should be made in the context of factors that would be used for any other pregnancy.

In the case of a second pregnancy, similar issues arise as with the first pregnancy; however, if HIV was discovered as a result of the first pregnancy, one has to consider whether the woman's sexual partner has been unlawfully put at risk. One also has to consider the effect on the mother of receiving temporary antiretroviral drug therapy, intended to reduce mother-to-child transmission, when she has no other opportunity of getting such treatment.

In Barbados, Kumar and St John (2001) studied 27 women who had additional pregnancies while they were known to be HIV-positive. It was reported that a third of the women did not know of the risk of transmission to the baby or that the AZT that they were given was to reduce the risk of transmission. Those figures suggest that either the women were lying to the investigators to remain sympathetic figures, or the counselling that was required for these women was particularly inept.

The infant

Should an HIV-positive premature infant be treated the same way as any other premature newborn? All infants should be treated in the same manner. One does not know whether the infant is infected, particularly when antiretroviral treatment has been given to reduce the risk of transmission of the virus.

A child's right to live in spite of its level of disability has been established in case law, even in cases of severe disability such as that caused by anencephaly. Closing the door on these infants not only ignores the possibility that they may not be infected but also denies them the opportunity to benefit from advances in care. It also denies the parents the child that they may have ardently desired.

Should the infant be ventilated if ventilators are scarce? All infants should be treated equally, and in situations where ventilation facilities are limited, protocols should be formulated for the guidance of staff.

What happens to the infant if the mother dies? The father or other relatives will be responsible for looking after the welfare of the child. If there are no relatives willing to bring up the child, the responsibility lies with the agency responsible for looking after the welfare of children, including arranging adoption or finding foster parents.

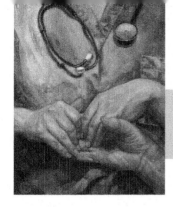

References

Botros, C.T. 2001. Clear and convincing evidence required to withdraw life-sustaining treatment in impaired but conscious patient. *Wendland v. Wendland. American Journal of Law and Medicine* 27:487–9.

Childs, M. 1995. Medicine and the law of manslaughter. *International Journal of the Medical and Dental Defence Unions* 9(3):36–9.

Ciesielski, C., D. Marianos, C-Y. Ou, R. Dumbaugh, J. Witte, R. Berkelman, B. Gooch et al. 1992. Transmission of human immunodeficiency virus in a dental practice. *Annals of Internal Medicine* 116:798–805.

Connor, S., and H. Fuenzalida-Puelma, eds. 1990. *Bioethics: Issues and Perspectives.* PAHO Scientific Publication No. 527.

Feinstein A. 1994. Clinical judgment revisited: The distraction of quantitative models. *Annals of Internal Medicine* 120:167–78.

Gracia, D. 1990. Medical bioethics. In Connor and Fuenzalida-Puelma 1990, 3–7.

Kumar, A., and A. St John. 2001. KAP among HIV-infected women with repeated childbirths in Barbados. *West Indian Medical Journal* 50 (Suppl. 2): 16.

Meisel, A. 1992. Retrospective on Cruzan. *Law, Medicine and Health Care* 20:340–53.

Miller, F. 1993. The concept of medically indicated treatment. *Journal of Medicine and Philosophy* 18:81–8.

Sass, H.-M. 1990. Bioethics: Its philosophical basis and application. In Connor and Fuenzalida-Puelma 1990, 18–23.

Suggested Readings

Daniels, N. Why justice is good for our health. In *Interfaces between Bioethics and the Empirical Social Sciences*, edited by F. Lolas and L. Agar, 37–52. PAHO/WHO, 2002.

Drane, J.F. What is bioethics? A history. In *Interfaces between Bioethics and the Empirical Social Sciences*, edited by F. Lolas and L. Agar, 15–32. PAHO/WHO, 2002.

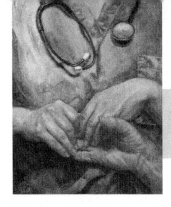

Index

CPSIA information can be obtained at www.ICGtesting.com
Printed in the USA
LVOW03s0224300615

444379LV00015B/139/P

9 789766 401641